SECRETS OF

NATURAL HEALING

WITH FOOD

SECRETS OF
NATURAL HEALING
WITH FOOD

WELLNESS AND
BODY CHEMISTRY

Nancy Appleton, Ph.D.

Rudra Press
PORTLAND, OREGON

Rudra Press
P.O. Box 13390
Portland, OR 97213
Telephone: (503) 235-0175
Telefax: (503) 235-0909

Compiled and edited by Aurelia Navarro
Book and cover design: Bill Stanton
Illustrations: Hannah Bonner
Cover photograph: Aaron Rezny

This book is not intended to replace expert medical advice. Because each person and situation is unique, the editor and publisher urge you to verify the appropriateness of any procedure or diet with your physician or other qualified health care professional.

Library of Congress Cataloging-in-Publication Data

Appleton, Nancy.
   The secrets of natural healing with food: wellness and body chemistry/Nancy Appleton.
       p.   cm.
   Includes bibliographical references and index.
   ISBN 0-915801-49-3
   1. Diet therapy.   2. Nutrition.   3. Homeostasis.   4. Food allergy — Diet therapy.
I. Title.
RC216.A45   1995
615.8'54—dc20   95-3820
                                                           CIP

00 99 98 97   10 9 8 7 6 5 4 3

FOREWORD

Nancy Appleton did it — she has written the book we've needed for a decade. As a physician practicing in wellness and preventive medicine since 1983, the body chemistry principles Dr. Appleton delineates in this book have become the basis of what I practice, teach, and use myself. It started in 1984, when a flyer from the Price-Pottenger Nutrition Foundation describing a weekend seminar on the body chemistry principle caught my eye. At that time, my patients were making good progress on the path to wellness, but it was clear there was still something missing. Could the body chemistry principle be the key?

After spending two days listening to Dr. Robert Bruce Pacetti reveal the secrets of balanced body chemistry, my life and my practice changed forever. My confusion about which dietary expert to believe was over — now I knew how to evaluate dietary information for each individual. Now I understood why people reacted so differently to the same foods, and why all nutritional counseling had to be personal. But even though I understood the body chemistry approach and found it simple and easy, I ran into plenty of difficulties in putting it in practice — for myself and for my patients.

And that's when Dr. Appleton came hundreds of miles to my rescue, bringing pots, pans, slicers, cutting boards, and her expertise to set up my "teaching kitchen." Here my patients could participate in preparing delicious meals and learn first hand how simple it can really be to eat healthfully. Dr. Appleton has continued to dedicate herself to sharing this message of health — often at her own expense — because it is a labor of love for her; she wants you to know how to be healthy and how to avoid needless suffering. This book you have in your hands will teach you how to overcome many unnecessary illnesses and discomforts if you are motivated to apply its principles in all the body chemistry arenas. With it, you can also pass a legacy of health to your children and grandchildren. The young are in desperate need of this information, because each successive generation's constitutions become weaker and weaker when their ancestors have lived constantly in upset body chemistry. Thus our children will develop degenerative diseases earlier in their lives than we did unless we share this message of health with them.

There are so many success stories in my practice. One mom came to me in despair because her 2 year old son was totally uncontrollable: he was literally climbing the walls, and he refused to eat anything but dairy products. After getting the family on Food Plan 3 and gradually eliminating dairy from the boy's diet, he calmed down into a very sweet child who would eat almost anything. Another two year old terror became calm and loving after removing sweets from her eating plan. My two daughters and I are all sugar sensitized (a common problem since approximately 30% of the population is sensitive and addicted to sugars). We each react a little differently: I become severely fatigued and irritable the day after eating sugar. My oldest daughter's brain goes fuzzy, and my youngest daughter gets happily higher than a kite at first, but pays for it with about four days of nothing but moan, groan, and complain when she hits withdrawal. Since she is naturally loving, talented, and a delightful person, well beyond her years in maturity, it is a shame to see her in the throes of the sugar rollercoaster. If your family is suffering through what seem like cause-less bouts of irritable, crabby, uncontrolled behavior, please read this book carefully — and start changing your life to a happy and healthy one.

Dr. Nancy Appleton did you a great favor in creating this book. It can guide you to personal responsibility for your own health. May you be greatly blessed as you use it to follow the road to optimal good health. Enjoy!

Bessie Jo Tillman, M.D.
President, Board of Directors
Price-Pottenger Nutrition Foundation

CONTENTS

HANDY REFERENCE TO

Quick Tips and Charts

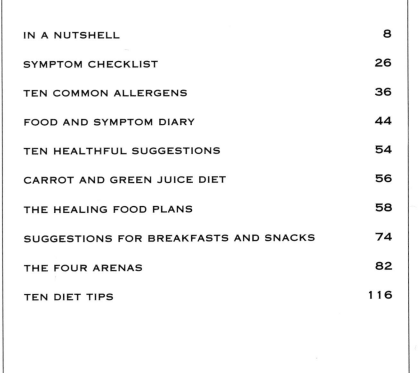

SECRETS OF
NATURAL HEALING
WITH FOOD

INTRODUCTION

Reclaim Your Right to Health

This book is about learning to reclaim your right of health and wellness. A balanced body chemistry is the secret ingredient. What you eat, how and where you live, how you feel and react, what you think, what you say, the chemicals in your environment — all of these things affect your body chemistry. When it is in a state of balance, this is called *homeostasis*, and it is your body's natural healing mode. Homeostasis is not a fixed or unchanging state; rather, it refers to your body's ability to respond to input — whether in the form of food, state of mind, drugs, environmental factors, or whatever — and *quickly* recover its state of balance. I have found, in my own experience and over and over with clients, that you can take charge of your health by learning how to stay in this natural healing mode.

The information in this book gives you everything you need in order to get your body into balance (homeostasis) and keep it there on a regular basis. When you are not able to maintain homeostasis on a regular basis, your body is more susceptible to disease, both infectious and degenerative. You influence your

3

body's chemistry through conscious and unconscious lifestyle choices — and the choice over which you have the most consistent and direct control is about what you eat.

The first 40 years of my life were filled with pain, both physical and mental. Like so many of us, I lived in a state somewhere between sickness and health. I wasn't sick enough for a hospital, but I was never exactly well, either. In fact, looking back, I realize that I didn't even know what "healthy" felt like. From a very young age I ate an incredible amount of sugar and chocolate. I was a National Junior Tennis Champion, so I played in many tournaments. If I won, I'd treat myself to two hot fudge sundaes. If I lost, I'd eat a whole bag of Oreo cookies to console myself. So whether I won or lost, my health was always the loser. My little body was filled with allergy: runny eyes and nose, scratchy throat, itchy ears, sneezing, and sinusitis. As I grew older, different symptoms appeared: arthritis, migraine headaches, canker sores, pneumonia (five times!), yeast infections, hypoglycemia, boils, fatigue, and continually falling asleep after eating. I needed 9 hours of sleep at night and a nap in the afternoon. I was taking pill after pill. The pills would relieve the symptoms temporarily but I never quite got well. Like most drugs, the pills I took for all those years only worked on the symptoms — the disease never went away.

It wasn't until I got frustrated enough to decide to take charge and learn how to create health for myself that I was able to turn my health around. Once I understood the principles of homeostatis, I was no longer a victim of unknown forces. I was able to take charge, I was able to heal myself and get well. I am healthier now at age 59 than I was at 18.

It has been my experience that we have tremendous power to affect our health, for good or ill, through what we *do*. And for me, the biggest changes had to do with what I ate. Sugar, caffeine, over-the-counter and prescription drugs, overheated fats, and overprocessed foods are all what I call "abusive foods" — and they can ruin our health. But the good news is that if we stop doing to the body what we did to make it sick, the body will heal itself. It really will. This book will show you how to stop doing to your body the things that make it ill...then the rest is up to you.

The fact that you are reading this now says that you are ready to take charge of your own health. Congratulations! I want to help you make healthy choices about what you put in your mouth, what comes out of your mouth, what you think and feel, what you allow into your environment, and what you choose to do. All of these make up your physical and mental well being and all are part of the balanced body

So let's get started! Remember that natural healing is a process of change and change takes time. This program is not a diet or regime that you do for a few weeks or months until you feel better or attain your ideal weight. This is a lifetime program. It is a process that can help keep you healthy for the rest of your life. Take the information in this book, add your own commitment and determination, and you too can create health for yourself.

CHAPTER 1

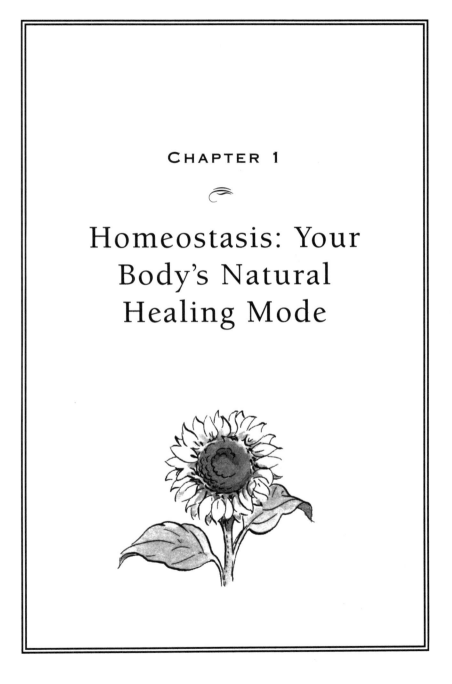

Homeostasis: Your Body's Natural Healing Mode

In a Nutshell

1. INFECTIOUS DISEASES, DEGENERATIVE DISEASES, AND ROBUST HEALTH ALL RESULT FROM THE CONDITION OF THE BODY'S CHEMISTRY. ALL FORMS OF HEALTH BREAKDOWNS RESULT FROM UPSET BODY CHEMISTRY.

2. THROUGH MANY LIFESTYLE INDISCRETIONS, YOUR BODY'S CHEMISTRY CAN GO OUT OF BALANCE IN A MOMENT. DEPENDING ON YOUR ADAPTIVE ABILITIES, YOUR BODY'S CHEMISTRY CAN EITHER STAY UNBALANCED OR REBALANCE IN VARIOUS LENGTHS OF TIME.

3. THE MAGNITUDE OF ANY HEALTH BREAKDOWN IS DETERMINED BY THE DEGREE AND DURATION OF UNBALANCED BODY CHEMISTRY.

4. A BODY IN BALANCE (HOMEOSTASIS) IS IN ITS NATURAL HEALING MODE.

5. THE ONLY DIFFERENCE BETWEEN A WELL PERSON AND A PERSON WITH HEALTH BREAKDOWNS IS THAT THE WELL PERSON CAN STILL EFFICIENTLY BRING HIS OR HER BODY CHEMISTRY BACK INTO THE NATURAL HEALING MODE AFTER THE UNBALANCING EFFECTS OF LIFESTYLE INDISCRETIONS.

6. HOW YOUR BODY RESPONDS TO APPROPRIATE DOCTORING AFTER A HEALTH BREAKDOWN DEPENDS ON THE RESILIENCE OF YOUR BODY'S CHEMISTRY.

7. YOU ARE IN CONTROL OF YOUR BODY'S CHEMISTRY BALANCE THROUGH YOUR CONSCIOUS AND UNCONSCIOUS LIFESTYLE CHOICES.

8. THROUGH EDUCATION AND COMMITTED ACTION YOU CAN CONSCIOUSLY WORK TO KEEP YOUR BODY IN HOMEOSTASIS — ITS NATURAL HEALING MODE.

L et's start with a definition. According to Webster's Dictionary, homeostasis is: "the maintenance of normal internal stability in the organism by coordinated responses of the organ systems that automatically compensate for environmental changes."

For human beings, homeostasis commonly refers to the internal balance of the body's electro-magnetic and chemical systems. This balance permits and encourages proper performance of the internal functions necessary for growth, healing, and life itself. We have many homeostatic mechanisms in our body which help maintain this balance, and our state of health is directly related to the health of these mechanisms. Our body chemistry is wonderfully complex and highly inter-related. All of the systems of our body relate to each other in some way. There are backup systems, feedback loops, and precisely calibrated relationships that we are still learning about every day.

When our body chemistry is in balance, our glands secrete the right amount of hormones into the bloodstream at the right moment and our body works wonderfully well. The ovaries secrete the right amount of estrogen and progesterone. The right amount of insulin is secreted from the pancreas at the right time to maintain a normal blood sugar. The thyroid gland secretes the correct amount of thyroxine into the bloodstream to regulate the many metabolic functions such as growth, the way we process foods, and the way we use oxygen. When our bloodstream needs extra adrenaline due to distresses such as excess fatigue, heat, cold, or other environmental factors, our adrenal glands come to our defense.

But when our bodies become over-stressed, none of these mechanisms work at their best, and homeostasis becomes more and more difficult to maintain. Let's look at some of the major factors of body chemistry to get an overview of how balance is protected — and how it can get go wrong. As you read, remember — the information in this book will show you how to make conscious choices that will help your body stay in balance, all the time, for the rest of your life.

ENZYMES

Enzymes are the catalysts that drive many of the chemical reactions that keep our bodies functioning. There are two main classes of enzymes in our body: metabolic enzymes, which help run the body, and digestive enzymes, which help digest our food.

Metabolic Enzymes

Our bodies, organs, and tissues are run by metabolic enzymes. We are living bundles of enzymes. Enzymes reshape, restructure, and reform all the raw material we take in. These enzymes do the special work needed to run the heart, brain, lungs, kidney and other organs, and regulate their correct functioning. Enzyme deficiencies can cause many problems. For example, new research indicates it may be an enzyme deficiency that causes cataracts. Although thousands of enzymes and their reactions are known, many more reactions have been identified for which the enzymes responsible are not yet known. Hundreds of metabolic enzymes are necessary to carry on the work in the body — to repair damage and decay and to heal diseases. Most enzymes do not work efficiently without minerals in the right proportions.

Digestive Enzymes

Digestive enzymes help you digest your food. And it is at the level of digestive enzymes that we start to pay the price for upsetting our body chemistry — many of the health problems we suffer can be traced back to whether or not the body's minerals (and therefore, enzymes) are in balance so that the all-important function of food digestion and utilization of nutrients can take place properly. If our digestive enzymes are out of balance, we don't get the full benefit from our food — and our food itself can become toxic, causing allergic symptoms of all kinds.

MINERALS

Enzymes are dependent on minerals, yet when homeostasis cannot be maintained, one of the first things to go out of balance is the relationship between the minerals in our system. These mineral relationships are very precisely calibrated; it is easy to throw this complex system out of balance.

Mineral Wheel

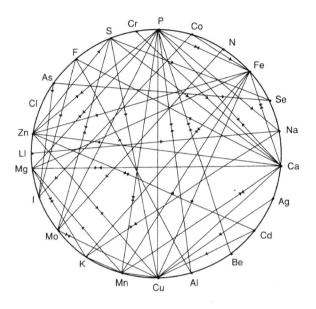

Source: Dr. Paul Eck, Analytical Research Labs, Inc., Phoenix, Arizona

Let's look at two important minerals that work in direct relationship to one another: calcium and phosphorus. These minerals work best in the bloodstream in a relationship of 2.5 parts calcium to 1 part phosphorus. Normally, the calcium level in the bloodstream is about 10 milligrams per deciliter, and the phosphorus level is 4 milligrams. This means that your ability to use the calcium in your system is *phosphorus dependent:* no matter how much calcium you have, you can only use it if there is enough phosphorus present to go with it.

Calcium and Phosphorus

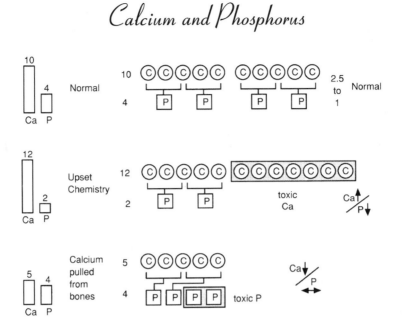

For example, if you upset your body chemistry and your phosphorus level drops to 2 mg per deciliter, rather than the normal 4, only 5 mg of calcium can be used by your body — the ratio must be 2.5 times as much calcium as phosphorus for the minerals to function optimally. Any additional calcium you may have will either be excreted in the urine or it may stay in the body and become what I call "toxic" — excess and non-functioning calcium that can cause a number of problems. For instance, the excess calcium may form hard deposits that irritate soft tissue. The plaque on your teeth that irriates your gums is an example of this. Or the toxic calcium can go to your joints and be a part of the arthritis process. In the arteries, toxic calcium can be a factor in arteriosclerosis. It can also contribute to kidney stones, bone spurs, gallstones, and cataracts.

But what if you have less calcium than you need? For example, if your calcium levels drop to 5 mg, then only 2 mg of phosphorus will be used. This could leave an excess of phosphorus, which also is either secreted or retained. If too much is retained, it, too, can become toxic. And that's not all! When there is an excess of phosphorus-to-calcium in your bloodstream, a message is sent to your body that calcium is needed — and your body will pull that calcium right out of your bones — causing osteoporosis, among other things.

It's a complex balancing act. These minerals do not work by themselves but work only in relation to each other. This means that the whole system can be immobilized if one of the minerals becomes deficient, even if the other minerals are present in the bloodstream. For instance, no matter how many units of calcium you have in the bloodstream, if you don't have enough phosphorus to make that 2.5:1 mixture, the calcium is not usable. So you can actually have an excess of calcium in your bloodstream and still be effectively deficient in usable calcium. This is why I advise everyone to stop drinking soft drinks — they all contain phosphorus, and tend to throw our calcium/phosphorus balance way out of line.

Copper and zinc are two other minerals that work in direct relation to each other. If the zinc becomes deficient, the copper can become toxic and vice versa. This is true of all the different minerals in the body; they all work in relation to one another. Therefore, directly or indirectly, all of the minerals can be affected if one of them becomes deficient or excessive.

Minerals are needed for many functions. Vitamins cannot function without minerals. Most enzymes cannot function without minerals. Many hormones need minerals to function, so that a lack of these minerals will lead to immobilization of vitamins, enzymes, and hormones.

HORMONES — THE ENDOCRINE SYSTEM

Our endocrine glands are very important in helping to maintain the balance of our body chemistry. These glands are scattered throughout the body. They secrete hormones into the bloodstream that help regulate the body chemistry. Each of these glands — adrenal, pancreas, thyroid, parathyroid, pituitary, hypothalamus, and gonads, among others — play an important part in maintaining homeostasis.

Endocrine System

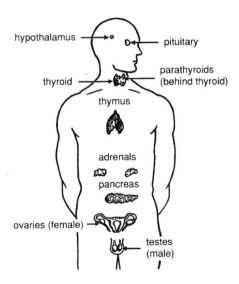

Source: *Healthy Bones*, Nancy Appleton. Avery Publishing Group, 1991. Used by permission.

The system has many built-in safeguards. If one of your glands is weak, other glands usually "kick in" to make up for the weak one. However, if you continually upset your body chemistry, the stronger glands have to kick in more and more often — and evenually they, too, become exhausted. For women, upset body chemistry combined with the natural hormonal shifts of puberty, menstruation, pregnancy, and menopause can have many adverse implications, including PMS, postmenopausal problems, osteoporosis, hypothyroidism, and exhausted adrenal glands. For all of us, an overworked endocrine system can have serious health implications.

Let me give you a few examples. Insulin is a hormone that is critical in the metabolism of sugar. Whenever we eat simple sugar, whether it's a candy bar, an apple, or sugar in your tea, our blood sugar (called glucose) goes up. When your body is healthy, just the right amount of insulin is secreted by the pancreas to bring the glucose back down. This is a normal homeostatic mechanism. In a diabetic, the insulin does not function properly and the diabetic must carefully control diet or take extra insulin to bring the sugar level down to normal and back to homeostasis. In diabetes, one of the body's homeostatic mechanisms is not functioning optimally.

Another mechanism is the ability of the adrenal glands to secrete adrenaline into the blood stream when our body faces a threat and needs an extra push to get us in motion quickly. When we were living in caves and were suddenly confronted with an angry bear, adrenaline would be secreted into the blood stream to give us added energy — and we would use up that energy either running or fighting. There are no bears chasing us today, yet the stresses of modern living still trigger that old adrenaline response. This is called the "fight or flight syndrome." But without bears to fight or run from, we don't "run off" the adrenaline, and it can cause a lot of problems. Modern life has many more opportunities for stress than our bodies were designed to handle. Many people live in such constant stress that they have exhausted their adrenal glands. A simple way to test your adrenals is to bend over and touch your toes. If you get lightheaded or a little dizzy when you get up, your adrenals are not functioning at their best.

HEALTH AND HOMEOSTASIS

The body always wants to come back into balance. All the systems fluctuate a little bit all the time. The glucose goes up and down a little, the phosphorus goes up and down a little in a narrow range and it's always trying to stay in the optimal range, where our body can function the best. A healthy person comes back to homeostasis easily and quickly. This is a good benchmark of health: how fast you can come back to balance after an "indiscretion" such as eating the wrong thing, or too much of the right thing, or eating when stressed. But a sick person doesn't come back to homeostasis quickly and sometimes doesn't come back at all.

The implications of upset body chemistry, a body out of homeostasis, are staggering. When the minerals change relationship to each other, vitamins, enzymes, and hormones are unable to function properly. This opens the door to infectious and degenerative diseases.

It all starts when the digestive process is compromised; for example, by eating excess sugar or other abusive foods. There is more detail on this process in Chapter 3, but to summarize, if your minerals are out of balance, some of the enzymes needed for digestion will be out of commission, and not all of your food will be fully digested. This means that not all of the food is broken down into its smallest, simplest form so that our body can utilize the essential nutrients in the food. Ideally, all of the protein we eat breaks down into amino acids, all of the carbohydrates break down into simple sugars, and all of the fats break down into fatty acids. Instead, some of the food remains in the intestines as large particles. You might think that they would simply be excreted via the feces but they are not. These large partially digested particles irritate the lining of the gastro-intestinal tract, and in time the cells on the sides of the gastro-intestinal tract widen and the partially digested foods gets into the bloodstream. This is called "the leaky gut syndrome." These large particles of semi-digested food in the bloodstream are the cause of food allergy symptoms and ultimately lead to an exhausted immune system.

How does this partially digested food affect our immune system? Our immune system treats these large chunks of semi-digested food as foreign matter. And since it is the job of the immune system to defend us from foreign particles, it tries to get this semi-digested food out of the body. But this system is usually meant to take only small amounts of undigested food out of the body, and then to take out bacteria, viruses, cancer cells, anything that does not belong there, out of the body. The immune system was not meant to come to our defense on a daily basis, meal after meal, week, month, year after year, decade after decade. The liver and other organs in the body become overworked and become exhausted. They cannot do the work needed to keep the body healthy. The body becomes toxic and problems develop. The immune system is exhausted. This exhaustion of the immune system leaves the door open for disease, both infectious and degenerative.

Once the immune system is compromised, we are vulnerable to those degenerative diseases that our genetic blueprint has left us open to — whether it be a form of cancer, or M.S., or any other disease. We are vulnerable also to infectious diseases: whatever bacteria or virus happens to be in our neighborhood, we will be more likely to get that illness. It's that simple. An imbalance of body chemistry, an upset in mineral relationships, leaves us vulnerable to disease of all kinds.

If we change our diet and stop eating abusive foods and foods that our individual bodies have abused (which are the food that cause us allergies) as well as reduce or remove the distress from our lives then our symptoms will diminish and we will be far less prone to diseases both infectious and degenerative. If colds and flu linger for more than a week, it is a clue that your immune system is not functioning as well as it could.

Since I have understood the principle of upset body chemistry and since I have balanced my body chemistry, I rarely get sick and when I do, my immune system is strong enough to help me get well quickly.

CHAPTER 2

Getting Started:
Listening to Your Body

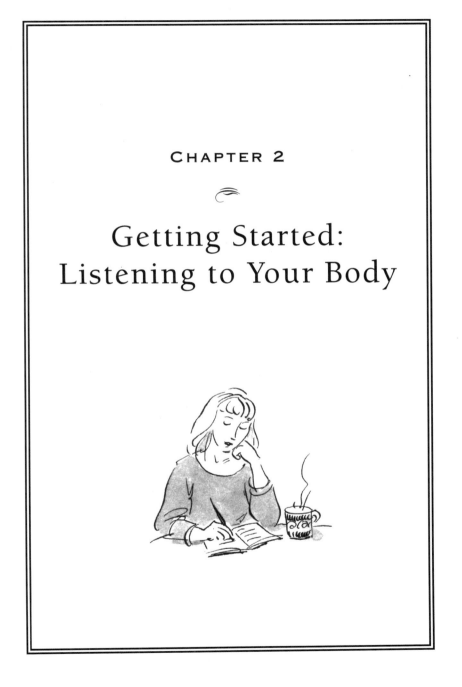

So You Don't Have Food Reactions

YOU MAY BE SURPRISED AT THE SORT OF SYMPTOMS THAT ARE FOOD RELATED. PEOPLE HAVE REPORTED IMPROVEMENT IN MANY OF THEIR SYMPTOMS AFTER LEARNING TO MANAGE BODY CHEMISTRY. HERE IS A PARTIAL LIST:

CANKER SORES

NAUSEA

ANXIETY

HEADACHE

CONFUSION

MUSCLE CRAMPS

ASTHMA

JOINT PAINS

ACNE

PMS SYNDROME

CHRONIC FATIGUE SYNDROME

What causes our body to lose its balance, to no longer be able to return to homeostasis quickly and efficiently?

Our twentieth century lifestyle is a major culprit in upsetting our body chemistry. Since the turn of the century, many things have changed in the way we live. Some of these so-called advances or advantages are not so advantageous to our body. For instance, at the turn of the century, we ate approximately 40 pounds of sugar per person per year. Today we eat 139 pounds of sugar per person per year. This sugar alone is an overwhelming insult to our body, to our immune system. Every time we eat sugar, we upset the delicate balance in our body.

Fast food restaurants have increased at a tremendous rate. Every year, MacDonalds sells billions of hamburgers, milkshakes, and french fries. The average adult eats out 11 times a week. Fast foods are usually fried foods, and therefore are notoriously high in the free radicals formed in the process of frying foods. The fats used for frying fast foods are often heated over and over and become rancid. These are the fats that clog the arteries, whether they be saturated or unsaturated. Stay away from all fried foods — they are killers.

At home, a lot of our food is packaged, processed, frozen, canned, overcooked, and filled with chemicals that didn't even exist 60 years ago.

Our bodies do not have the evolutionary mechanisms to digest these types of food. Our ability to change our world is moving much faster than our biological ability to adapt to change. Our bodies are still "pre-set" to digest the simple, fresh foods of earlier generations.

Prescription and over-the-counter drugs have increased at alarming rates. People go to doctors looking for the magic pill. The doctors listen to the patient's symptoms and prescribe a pill. The pill takes the symptoms away for a while, but the symptoms come back if the person stops taking the pill. The doctor never says, "I wonder what you could be doing to cause the problem, the headache, the fatigue, etc?" People really don't want to hear that they are doing something to cause these problems. We want a magic pill whether it's from a doctor and called tetracycline or Valium or from a practitioner in the nutritional field and called a vitamin, mineral, or enzyme. None of these magic pills or potions will work as long as we are upsetting our body chemistry.

HOW DO YOU KNOW?

How do you know whether your body is in homeostasis or not? Start listening to your body. This is the most important step. Your body gives you signals all the time that all is not well. We have not learned to listen to our body and read the signals. Chances are you are reading this book now because you have symptoms that just won't go away — and your doctor hasn't been able to help you. I believe that we can go through life with a minimum of diseases. It is up to each of us to keep our body in homeo-stasis and healthy. Although statistics show that one out of two of us will die of heart disease; one out of three will create cancer; one out of five of us will develop diabetes; and one out of six will get diagnosable mental illnesses, I don't think that this is necessary. I think that all of us can die of old age without these symptoms. Our hearts can just stop beating.

Here is a sample of some of the signals that all is not well within. Please check with your personal physician first if you have any of these symptoms, and assure yourself that they are not part of a larger disease picture. I have divided symptoms into five categories: gastrointestinal, central nervous system, musculoskeletal, respiratory, and miscellaneous. Use the checklist on the following pages to pinpoint your individual responses. I encourage you to work through the checklist today (using the first column) — and then come back to it in six to eight weeks after you have started improving your body chemistry. If you follow the guidelines in Chapter 4 carefully, I know you will see a great difference!

Symptom Checklist

Check off any symptoms you have now, then look at the Four Arenas (p. 82) and Food Plans (p. 58). Change what you need to in your lifestyle for two months and then go through the list again.

Gastrointestinal

9/16 — 11/16

__ anorexia   __ nervous stomach

__ binge eating   __ irritable colon

✓ bloating   __ diarrhea

__ canker sores   ✓ gas

__ excessive belching   ✓ constipation

__ indigestion   __ hungry (between meals)

__ nausea   __ vomiting

Central Nervous

✓ nervousness   ✓ headache

✓ fatigue   ✓ hostility

✓ anxiety   ✓ irritability

__ depression   __ mood change

__ hyperactivity   ✓ insomnia

__ confusion   __ high blood pressure

✓ dizziness   ? ✓ low blood pressure

✓ drowsiness   __ fullness of head

Musculoskeletal-Respiratory

__ muscle aches   __ hay fever

__ muscle cramps   __ palpitations

__ swelling   __ sinusitis

✓ stiffness   __ dark circles under eyes

__ irregular heartbeat   __ runny nose

__ increased heartbeat   __ scratchy throat

__ congestion in chest   __ itchy ears

__ asthma   __ joint pains

Skin

__ hives   __ edema

__ rash   __ eczema

__ acne   __ unusual skin pallor

__ psoriasis

Gynecological

__ vaginal discharge

__ vaginal itching

__ PMS Syndrome

__ menopausal symptoms

__ menstrual cramps

__ swollen breast(s)

__ lumps in breast(s)

Other

__ *Candida Albicans*

__ Epstein Barr Virus

__ Chronic Fatigue

__ water retention

✓ hyperglycemia

__ hypoglycemia

If you have checked any of these symptoms — and you have been assured by your personal physician that they are not symptoms of any underlying disease that requires treatment — then these are symptoms that say your body is not in homeostasis or balance. Some of the most common symptoms are headache, fatigue, joint pain, lower back pain, and falling asleep after meals. You know that 3 o'clock coma you fall into every afternoon at work? It could just be the bread in your lunch!

And how about the question of "How long do you stay out of balance, how long does it last?" Well, that depends on each individual. It can be affected by how much stress you had in the last couple of days, by whether you've had exercise, how old you are, how much you have abused your body, if you have been overeating, and if you have recently eaten abusive foods such as sugar, alcohol, caffeine, fried foods, or food to which you are allergic.

Another factor involved is your genetic blueprint. It depends on how strong your glands were when you were born as to how fast they come back to homeostasis and how well they can function. You might be born with some genetically weak glands. That in itself doesn't matter much. It just means that you will have a certain profile. But when you start abusing your body with sugar and stress, those glands that were not born very strong become weaker and can become a problem.

We'll go into more detail in Chapter 4, but just for starters, plan to try a healing food plan for at least one month, and preferably two months, before you decide whether it is going to work for you. After years of abuse and forced loss of balance, it will take time for your body to detoxify and readjust to new inputs.

STRESS, HOMEOSTASIS, AND THE MIND/BODY CONNECTION

Stress plays such an important part in our body chemistry, in homeostasis. In this life I have chosen to be a nutritionist, but in my next life, I think I will be a therapist to help people deal with their psychological problems.

Early in my research career, I wanted to test whether stress would upset the body chemistry. To find this out, I asked some volunteers to come to the lab while fasting. They had not eaten for 12 hours. I took their blood to find out what their fasting calcium and phosphorus ratio was. Then I needed to "distress" them to measure the difference. I did this by immersing one of their hands in ice water for one minute. Then I took their blood again to see if it had changed. I took blood every hour for four hours to see when the minerals would come back to balance. I found that the phosphorus became depleted and, of course, all of the minerals changed relationships to each other and became depleted and/or toxic. The ice water was a physical stress, but mental distress does the same thing.

Now when I speak of stress, I distinguish it from distress. We all have stress, we have parents and children, we all drive on freeways, we all have jobs, most of us have bosses and that's stress, but it's not life situations that cause the distress. It's how we deal with the stress that determines whether it will become distress.

TRY THIS EXPERIMENT...

Picture yourself walking outside into a grove of lemon trees. Look at those big yellow lemons on the trees. Smell their sharp, clean scent. Take one lemon and pull it off the tree and smell it. Now I want you to cut it in half and smell the inside of the lemon. Now lick it — taste the juice from the cut half. And now, take a big bite into the lemon.

I imagine by now you are salivating or close to it. This is the power of thought! In this case it was the thought of a lemon, something pleasant, something benign. But there are other thoughts: fearful thoughts, depressed thoughts, thoughts that put you in rage, thoughts of judgment and vengeance. All of those thoughts can upset your body chemistry. You are not only responsible for what you put in your mouth and what comes out of your mouth, but you are also responsible for what you think and how you feel!

We know instinctively that stress plays an important role in the disease process. Scientific studies back up our intuition. One study measured the effectiveness of a certain type of cell within the immune system, the phagocyte. The phagocyte is a type of white blood cell that functions like a "PacMan" of the body — its job is to gobble up intruders, foreign objects, unfamiliar cells. Normally each phagocyte can gobble up 16 foreign invaders. This is called the phagocyte index. This study measured that index when a person was under stress and found that the phagocyte's capacity to consume foreign invaders dropped dramatically.

Dr. Arthur Kaslow writes in his book, *Freedom From Chronic Disease*, that most chronic and degenerative diseases stem from the over-stimulation of the lymphocytes in a certain target area of the body. What name we call it just depends on what area of the body becomes inflamed — if it's the joints, we call it arthritis, if it's in the heart or circulatory system, we call them cardiovascular disorders, and so on. He says that it may well be that no specific "cause" will ever be identified for these chronic ailments. I feel that Kaslow is correct. None will be identified. We just need to stop upsetting our body chemistry — that is the cause.

Few have understood what exactly goes on in the body when our immune system is depressed. Now you know that the first thing that happens is the minerals become upset and then the chain of events continues. You could be on the best diet in the world and yet if you are under distress you would upset your body chemistry and would not be able to fully digest that food. The nutrients would be less available to the cells, and the partially digested particles could become "toxic," and you could get symptoms such as headaches, joint pains, fatigue, nausea or bloating. Or, if you are fortunate and have a resilient immune system, you may get no symptoms at all. When there are symptoms, the medical community tends to treat the result rather than the cause — with pain medication, tranquilizers, stimulants, anti-depressants, muscle relaxants, anti-convulsants, diuretics, nutrients and even the surgical removal of symptom-producing tissue. Of course, the best cure is just withdrawal. I'll say it again, because it is so important: Stop doing to the body what you did to make it sick and the body will heal itself.

It has been over 15 years since I started on this path to health. The first year was a process of ups and downs. I would learn, then make a mistake and then have to relearn. The process is evolutionary, not revolutionary. We are evolving human beings and change takes time. Make a commitment to yourself today to give yourself the time for this change. Promise to give yourself eight weeks to test a new way of eating and living that could just make you well!

The following chapters will tell you more about the role of food in the balanced body and most importantly will give you the simple food plans that you can use to put your body in its natural healing mode — and let the body heal itself.

CHAPTER 3

What's Food Got To Do With It?

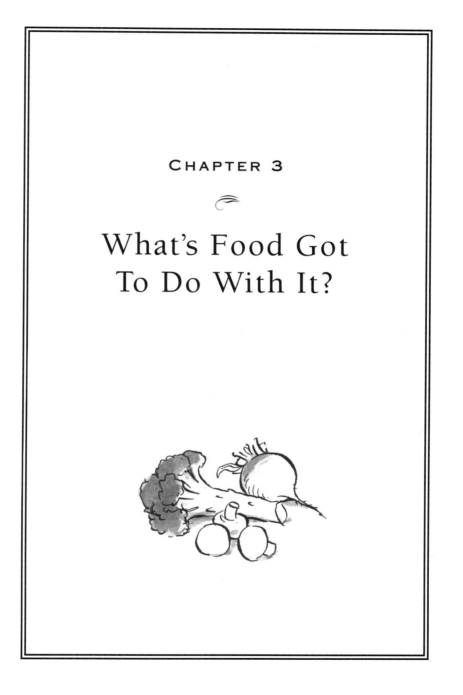

Ten Common Allergens

IF YOU HAVE SYMPTOMS THAT YOU THINK MIGHT BE FOOD RELATED BUT WANT PROOF, TRY ELIMINATING THESE FOODS FOR 2 MONTHS. THIS IS THE ESSENCE OF FOOD PLAN 3, THE MAXIMUM HEALING FOOD PLAN DESCRIBED IN CHAPTER 4. MANY PEOPLE HAVE BEEN AMAZED AT HOW MUCH BETTER THEY FEEL. THEN USE THE FOOD/SYMPTOM DIARY TO HELP PINPOINT YOUR INDIVIDUAL ALLERGIES AND SENSITIVITIES.

1. SUGAR: TABLE SUGAR (SUCROSE), GLUCOSE, FRUCTOSE, HONEY, MAPLE SUGAR, CORN SYRUP, CORN SWEETENER, RAW SUGAR, INVERT SUGAR, TURBINADO SUGAR, BROWN SUGAR, RICE SYRUP, DEXTROSE, DEXTRINE, BARLEY MALT.

2. MILK PRODUCTS: MILK, CHEESE, COTTAGE CHEESE, CREAMED CHEESE, YOGURT, CREAM, SOUR CREAM.

3. KOLA FAMILY: CHOCOLATE AND COLA ARE THE USUAL SOURCES.

4. WHEAT: BREAD, PASTA, CAKES, COOKIES, CRACKERS, DOUGHNUTS.

5. YEAST: BAKER'S YEAST AND BREWER'S YEAST.

6. ALCOHOL: BEER, WINE, AND HARD LIQUOR.

7. CORN: CORN ON THE COB, CORN SYRUP, CORN SWEETENER, DEXTROSE, DEXTRINE.

8. EGG: EGG WHITE AND/OR EGG YOLK.

9. PEANUT: RAW, ROASTED, PEANUT BUTTER.

10. CITRUS FRUITS: ORANGES, MANDARIN ORANGES, TANGERINES, GRAPEFRUIT.

Many of us have food allergies today. Some people are lactose intolerant and have to avoid dairy products. Some people are allergic to other common foods, others are allergic to molds or pollens — and some lucky individuals have no allergies at all. It may seem very confusing, since allergies are so particular to each individual — the healthiest foods can trigger an allergic reaction in some people. The answer to why some people are allergic and others are not has to do with upset body chemistry — a lack of balance. People can be out of balance due to stress, other life style factors, excess sugar, rancid fats — a few are even born with upset body chemistry.

In fact, each one of us has foods to which we react but if we have a healthy body the reaction will be slight and the body will come back to homeostasis or balance quickly. That is what health is: a quick rebalancing of the body. A sick person has a difficult time regaining and maintaining homeostasis. When we have lots of symptoms, the body does not come back to balance for a long time — and sometimes not at all. The homeostatic mechanism is not working correctly and the degenerative disease process is starting.

SENSITIVITY OR ALLERGY?

The word sensitivity might be a better word than allergy. In classical medical language, an allergy is a reaction that is "IgE mediated." Let me explain. We all have antibodies which are white blood cells and part of our immune system, also called immunoglobulins, abbreviated as "Ig". There are several different kinds of immunoglobulins, each denoted by a different ending letter: IgG, IgE, IgA, IgD and IgM. Classical allergists believe that the only way to test an allergy is if it is "IgE mediated" — that is, if the allergen reacts to immunoglobulin E. Some allergists are also testing for IgG reactions. My own research indicates that undigested food can react to any one of the other immunoglobulins — IgA, IgD, or IgM — as well as other parts of the immune system, but this is still not recognized by classical allergists, therefore the word sensitivity is a better choice. If your body shows symptoms after you eat, you are sensitive to that food whether it is IgE mediated or not. That food should be removed from your diet for a time to give your immune system a chance to strengthen itself. Then it can defend you from the foreign invaders that it is supposed to defend you against, such as bacteria, viruses, cancer cells, AIDS, and others. It will not waste its time and energy defending you from the food you eat every day.

HOW DO ALLERGIES DEVELOP?

As we have shown, when you are upsetting your body chemistry, your minerals change relation to each other. When you upset this delicate balance in the body, other body functions become impaired. The enzymes cannot function as well because enzymes are mineral dependent. We have many, many enzyme systems in our body and the functioning of the enzymes depends on there being enough minerals in the right relationship. Otherwise, the enzymes cannot function properly and the food we eat does not get thoroughly digested.

Incompletely digested food can get into the bloodstream, but its nutrients cannot be utilized by the cells. These large semi-digested particles are one form of food allergy and can cause havoc in the body. These particles can go to the brain and cause headaches, fatigue, or depression. They can go to the joints and cause pain. They can go to the arms and legs and cause swelling or to anywhere in the body and cause a problem. Food allergy can cause many symptoms in addition to the usual runny nose, weepy eyes, and itchy throat, as you have seen from the symptom checklist on page 26.

To further complicate matters, you might not have any symptoms until 6 or even 48 hours after you eat a food — you may never have connected your symptom with a food you ate the day before. When you have an immediate reaction, it's easy to figure out: You eat a piece of shrimp, and you break out in a rash or get hot all over or have some other symptom. Or you eat some peanut butter and your stomach gets crampy. Those allergies are easy; if that food is eliminated, the symptoms do not happen again. It's the delayed reactions that cause trouble for most of us. And remember, "delayed" can mean anywhere from 6 to 48 hours after you ate the food. These reactions are quite difficult to track down because you will have eaten a variety of food during that time. It is not easy to know which food caused the problem or even correlate the problem to a food, because by the time your joints start hurting or you get a migraine headache, it could be a full day after you ate the problem food.

There are other ways that food can affect your balance. Allergy can be the result of overeating a good thing, eating good things together with bad things or eating good things while we are in a bad frame of mind, to name a few possibilities.

For example, if you eat too much of any specific food at one sitting, you can exhaust the enzymes needed to digest that food. For instance, even though mashed potatoes are a healthy food, it is difficult for a person who has upset body chemistry to sit down and eat a mound of them. We only have so many enzymes and when we use them up — that's it. The food just doesn't digest. Give your enzymes a chance to rejuvenate by eating less of any one food and more variety at each meal.

Here's another example. Let's say you have a cheeseburger and a coke for lunch. Of course the coke has a lot of sugar in it, and sugar is almost always a trigger for loss of balance, because of its heavy demands on our endocrine, mineral, and enzyme systems. So, the sugar upsets your chemical balance, and your lunch is not completely digested. Now you have large particles of partially digested food that get into your bloodstream but cannot be utilized by the cells. One result of this kind of upset is that the body identifies the components of that food as potential allergens. So as a result of that cheeseburger and coke, you may end up with an allergy to wheat or yeast or eggs or tomato or any other individual food that was in that cheeseburger.

Overloading

At the time of the year when the pollens are out I used to have many allergies. I would get a runny nose and weepy eyes. Now that I am not abusing my body on a daily basis with foods to which I react, I do not have those seasonal allergies. What does happen though is that if I drink orange juice during that time, I sneeze more and my eyes run. I seem to react to the orange juice only during the seasonal pollen time.

This is an example of overdosing or overloading. Your immune system can be challenged by a variety of things, and when there are too many challenges at once, your immune system can become overloaded and hyper-reactive. In other words, things that you normally would not react to can become a problem at that time. Sometimes this happens when you are sick, which is why I advise you to eat sparingly when you are ill.

There are a couple of other items which cause food allergies and/or inhalant allergies. One of these is overcooking, which can denature the protein. Overcooked foods include TV dinners, homogenized dairy products, fried foods, and processed food that comes from the grocer in boxes, like cake mixes and pizza. I will talk more about the cooking and preparation of food in Chapter 4. Anything that causes upset body chemistry can cause allergy.

We talked a little about stress and distress in Chapter 2. It must be mentioned again here, because stress can cause allergies. You might not have put anything you are allergic to in your mouth or stomach but if you become distressed through anger, rage, depression, anxiety, or holding judgments against others and then eat, the food will not digest; it will just become an allergy for you. If you feel stressed, do not sit down to a meal, just push the food away and do whatever you need to do to put your body back in homeostasis. You could listen to an inspirational tape, meditate, pray, take a walk, write in your journal, practice yoga — do whatever it takes to break the hold of stress on your body before you eat or that food can become an allergen.

Remember there is no instant stress reduction just like there are no instant cures. On a daily basis you need to change your habits: change the way you eat and change the way you look at the world.

BE YOUR OWN "ALLERGY DETECTIVE"

So how can you learn which foods are problems for you? The best way is to become your own "allergy detective." Keep careful track of everything you eat and observe your responses. One of the best ways is by keeping a diary of everything you eat and all of your symptoms for two or three weeks. Over that period of time, patterns will emerge — and some of them will surprise you! Then, keep track of your progress through this program in the same diary. A sample diary page is shown on page 44. Use any small notebook that you can keep in your pocket or pocketbook. Every day, list everything you eat and then note any symptoms that you have. Remember that symptoms can be delayed for up to 48 hours. (And also remember that this is a first step. Some critical chemical imbalances may not produce any obvious symptoms. To learn about these, you need to use the Body Chemistry Kit, described on page 168.)

Before I became well, many foods bothered me. If I ate yeast my ankles would get swollen the next day and this swelling would last for about 24 hours. If I drank orange juice I started sneezing immediately. Grapefruit juice did the same thing. Baking powder made my right eye run. It is interesting that yeast never made me sneeze and grapefruit juice didn't make my eyes run. There were very specific reactions for the different foods. Your reactions may be very different. I had both immediate and delayed reactions. If you eliminate the food you react to for about two months, the allergy to that food will usually go away. But some allergies will take longer and some may never go away; you may simply need to learn to live without those foods, but these are few.

Plan on repeating this detective process from time to time, because your sensitivities will change over time, especially if you continue to upset your body chemistry by what you eat, think, do, or say.

ALLERGY VS ALLERGY-ADDICTED

When you have finished a meal, you should feel no better or no worse. You should feel just the same. If you feel better you are allergy-addicted to the food, if you feel worse you are just plain allergic to the food. We all know people who wake up saying, "I just have to have that cup of coffee." Well, they do feel better when they drink that cup of coffee — they do for a while — but then their blood sugar level drops, they crave that food or drink again and they have to have another cup of coffee or eat something sweet to keep themselves high. Those people are allergic to the food and they are addicted to the food also. Because even if

Food and Symptom Diary

DATE/TIME	FOOD	SYMPTOM
3/11 8 AM	1 BANANA	
	1 GLASS O.J.	
	CHEERIOS	
9 AM		BLOATED

you feel better after you have eaten a food, you will only feel better for a short period of time. How much food you eat, how much you are addicted to it, and your own biological makeup determine how long you feel better, but the addiction cycle is clear: first you actually do feel better but then you start to feel worse — just like a drug or alcohol addict does. When you start to feel worse you look again for that food hoping that it will pick you up — and over time you start to need more and more: more coffee, more sugar, and so on and on. This is allergy-addiction. As you can imagine, this cycle has a lot of bad implications for weight loss. Many life-long (and ultimately unsuccessful) dieters have found that their "will power" magically increased if they just cut out the foods that threw them into this allergy-addiction cycle. The healing food plans in Chapter 4 make the best diet for everyone — whether you are overweight, underweight, or just right. I'll talk more specifically about weight loss in Chapter 6.

If you find that you tend to time your snacks and meals so that you are always putting something in your mouth to feed that addiction, you may be not only allergic to the food, you are also addicted to it. Our bodies learn to adapt to this cycle at first, but eventually the body can no longer adapt; it becomes exhausted and that's when the degenerative disease process starts.

This whole cycle of peak and crash, peak and crash is very common. When I lecture I would much rather give my talks before lunch or before dinner because right after meals, all the people who are allergic or allergy-addicted to their routine foods will start to fall asleep. Fatigue is a very common allergic reaction. I can look around an audience and see right away who has been eating sugar and who is allergic to food, just by the fact that they are falling asleep. Not everyone reacts to food allergy with sleepiness, but it certainly happens to a lot of people — and they're the ones who start to fall asleep right in front of my eyes. The sleepyheads in the audience are a great visual aid for me.

COMMON ALLERGENS

Lets look at the ten food groups that are the most common causes of allergy. Take another look at the list at the beginning of this chapter. You may find this list surprising, since it includes so many foods we know to be of high nutritional quality. As you will see, it is another consequence of our 20th century lifestyle that so many of these fine foods have become allergens for so many of us.

After sugar, milk products are number two on the "common food allergy" list. Why? Milk is usually pasteurized, a process that involves heating to a very high temperature. The problem is that pasteurized milk is heated past what is called its "heat labile" point — the point at which it changes its chemical configuration. Any food can be cooked past this "heat labile" point and become a problem for us to digest. This is one of the problems with fried foods, and is also the reason why I suggest you eat as many foods as possible raw or lightly steamed. Food is made up of four major elements — nitrogen, oxygen, carbon, and hydrogen — along with trace minerals. Different foods have different combinations of those elements. We have evolved from early man with enzymes to digest foods in certain configurations. Modern food processing has brought massive changes to our food in the last fifty or so years — and we do not have the evolutionary enzymes to digest these new products.

We also eat a large percentage of our milk products with sugar: chocolate milk, milkshakes, ice cream, flavored yogurt, cheesecake, eggnog, breakfast cereal — it is a long list! So, there are many ways in which we have abused that good cow's milk — and many people are unable to digest cow's milk as a result.

Third on the list of common foods that many of us are allergic to is wheat. Wheat, the staff of life, is certainly not an abusive food, but we have abused it — first of all by making it into white flour by bleaching it and stripping it of many of its nutrients. Then let's say we make donuts: we add sugar to it and then we deep fry it. Adding sugar to the white flour and then deep frying it, what could be worse? We make it into Danish pastries, we make it into cakes and cookies, and we eat it over and over again. Wheat is in all of our fast foods. So we have abused that lovely wheat, and many of us have become allergic to it.

Another food that we have abused is yeast, and many of us are allergic to it as well. We have abused yeast by eating it as bread that we have to cook for a long time in the oven, and we have used our yeast with sugar.

Many of us are also allergic to corn. Yes, we can become allergic to corn on the cob, but the corn on the cob is not what started the allergy. It is because food producers have taken that corn and refined it into corn syrup or corn sweetener and used it in many of our processed foods. Corn syrup is much cheaper than beet or cane syrup, so rather than using the beet or the cane for sugars today in processed foods, they're using corn. So again we have abused that corn by making it into a sweetener and many of us have become allergic to it. Corn sweeteners are used in ketchup, in cranberry sauce, in most processed foods today. It may be called corn syrup or corn sweetener, or it may be called dextrose or dextrine. Read your labels and you will be surprised how much it is used.

Many of us also react to eggs. The good old American breakfast of orange juice, eggs, bacon, and toast is quite difficult to digest. Eggs, bacon, and toast have lots of protein. But when you eat your protein with orange juice, which is a simple sugar, it is more difficult to digest. Protein starts its digestion in the stomach, where it requires an acid state. So, when you eat protein, hydrochloric acid is secreted from the lining of the gastrointestinal tract. But when you add the orange juice, the protein has a harder time being digested because the fruit juice changes the acid state of the stomach into an alkaline state. So, perhaps the reason so many of us are allergic to eggs is because we've been eating them with orange juice in the morning as well as in cakes and cookies and in many sweet morsels such as custards and cheese cakes.

Aspirin also has a role in allergy. Research from various sources shows that aspirin has the ability to increase the permeability of the gastric mucosa, the stomach lining, for up to thirty minutes after ingestion. This means that any incompletely digested food that is in the stomach when we take aspirin can sneak into the bloodstream more easily because of the increased permeability of the lining. And we already know that these large articles of semi-digested food become a food allergy with all of the problems that go with allergy. If you know that you are allergic to a food and you eat it and take an aspirin at the same time you could provoke a far greater reaction than if you had eaten the allergic food without the aspirin. There are a lot of other problems with aspirin as well. I suggest that you find out why you need the aspirin, and do what you can to change the part of your lifestyle that is causing the problem, so you will not need the aspirin.

≈

INHALANTS, ENVIRONMENTALS, AND FOOD ALLERGIES

Why is it that some people sneeze at hibiscus, others feel faint at the gas pump, and others become nauseated at the smell of food frying? Still others have no inhalant allergies at all. At certain times of the year, allergies for some are worse than at other times of the year. People who have environmental allergies may have problems when the hot winds come to town or when they ride a horse; petting a cat can become a problem for some, while reading a newspaper can cause a feeling of weakness in others, certain flowers can give some of us a runny nose, and the list goes on. Whether they know it or believe it, these people have food allergies. Once they deal with the food allergies, the environmental allergies go away. Once they have stopped upsetting their body with foods to which they react, their immune system becomes strong and they are able to deal with the inhalant allergies. People with strong immune systems do not have allergies. If you do have inhalant allergies, get on Food Plan 3, the maximum healing food plan, as described in Chapter 4. You will be amazed that your inhalant allergies will go away.

Some people can be called "universal reactors." Because they have a suppressed immune system, they develop allergies to just about everything in their environment: chemicals, foods, and inhalants (dust, molds and pollens). Immune systems can be congenitally weak, as we have discussed, or can become compromised in a variety of ways, including viral infections, poor eating habits, stress, and chronic exposure to environmental chemical pollutants that first weaken the immune system.

These people must change their lifestyle completely in order to stop upsetting their body chemistry. There is a plan outlined in Chapter 6. It is centered, again, on Food Plan 3 for maximum healing, but it also addresses all four arenas of lifestyle. This is not easy, but the payoff is worth it.

As you have seen, it is not one thing that throws the body out of balance, it is a whole lot of things. The combination of a little stress, a little sugar, an order of French fried potatoes, and a fried hamburger might be too much for your body, and an allergic reaction could occur.

The best diet for all people consists of small amounts of protein and a plentiful variety of vegetables, potatoes, and beans. You can eat every 2 hours if necessary. People who have symptoms have lost the ability to come back to balance quickly and have enzymes that do not function optimally. They need to eat small amounts of food and a good variety. When you eat a variety of foods you get a variety of minerals, and you pull from a variety of enzyme systems to digest those foods — so hopefully you won't exhaust your enzyme supply. Potatoes only need a few enzymes and if you eat a large mound you are more likely to run out of enzymes for those potatoes than if you eat a small amount from a variety of foods. Notice I said a small amount. You could eat a good variety of food, but if you eat too much of all of them, you will also exhaust your enzymes. So eating too much of one or eating too much of a variety can both be detrimental to your health.

The only way to bring the body back to balance is to stop upsetting it. Taking extra minerals will not bring the minerals back to balance. You might sit down and have a good meal that supplies all the vitamins and minerals researchers say you should have each day, making sure that you get a lot of vegetables, some protein, some beans, maybe some potatoes, small amounts of a variety of foods. You must stop eating there. You can't say to yourself, "since I've been so good, I will treat myself to a hot fudge sundae for dessert." The nutrients you put into your body with the vegetable and protein will not be properly utilized when you eat the hot fudge sundae, because it upsets your body chemistry. When you take 600 mg of calcium in the form of a milkshake which has about 8 teaspoons of sugar, or in the form of fruit yogurt which has 7 teaspoons of sugar or honey, you will not be able to metabolize all the calcium because the sugar or honey so upsets the body chemistry that the calcium cannot function. You have literally put all those good nutrients in your mouth but they cannot function in your body.

Start with eliminating the most common "unbalancing" foods, and then carefully observe your individual reactions, your personal sensitivities. Follow the simple guidelines in the next chapter, and re-claim your right to health. It requires some effort, some planning, and a healthy dose of commitment, but the reward is great. I believe so strongly in this theory of homeostasis and balanced chemistry because it has changed my life so completely — and I want to share this great good fortune with each of you. Let's get going!

CHAPTER **4**

Taking Charge:
The Healing Food Plans

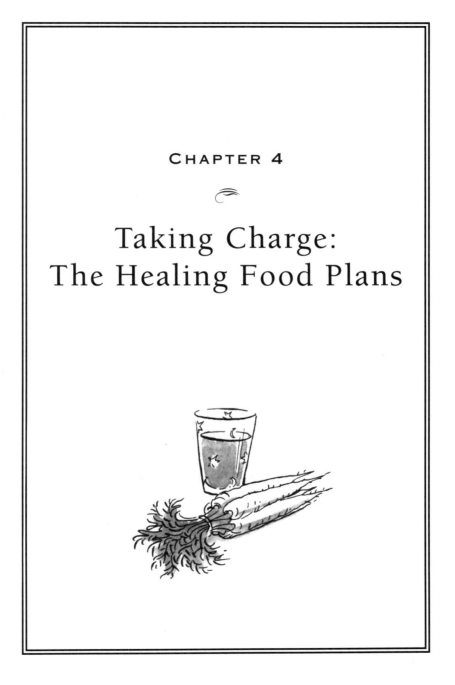

10 Healthful Suggestions

1. Chew each mouthful of food at least 20-28 times.

2. Only drink liquid when there is no food in your mouth, so that you don't swallow the food undigested.

3. Drink most of your liquids between meals.

4. Consume only portions you feel you can safely digest.

5. When you are emotionally upset or disturbed, eat smaller portions and chew more thoroughly.

6. Undercook rather than overcook your food. This means lightly steam your vegetables and cook beans and proteins at low temperatures.

7. Broil, bake, steam, stir fry or slow-cook your food rather than fry it.

8. The more raw food you eat, the better.

9. Eat frequent small meals rather than fewer large meals.

10. Examine each meal and snack from the viewpoint, "Does any part of this meal upset my body chemistry and promote the disease process?"

On the next several pages, you will find a complete listing of three different food plans. In each food plan, you have lots of variety to choose from, delicious food you can enjoy as your body is allowed to rest and begin the healing process. Foods are listed in five major categories, with subheadings in each category. The more strictly you adhere to the food plans — the fewer substitutions and little moments of "cheating" — the faster you will get well and the more dramatic that improvement will be.

But it is entirely up to you. There are several ways you can use the information in these food plans. For instance, I feel strongly that *everyone* should avoid all the substances in Category V and Category VI. If you feel that you are generally healthy and just want to make sure you stay that way, I recommend Food Plan 1, for maintaining health. Start by filling out the Symptom Checklist on page 26. Then just avoid all the substances in Categories IV and V for seven days and re-work the Checklist. If there is not a significant improvement, go on to Food Plan 2, and so on. Or, if you know you need maximum healing, go directly to Food Plan 3.

Whichever way you proceed, remember there are at least two steps to finding the right foods for you. First, you need to find the right Food Plan. Second, you have to customize that plan by finding which foods are your individual allergens. For this, use your Food and Symptom Diary. When testing a food or food group, first make sure you have been eating simply for at least seven days so your digestive system is rested and relatively balanced. Then add just one food or food group for three days, and carefully observe and record your symptoms. You need to allow three days so that delayed reactions have a chance to show themselves.

How long does it take for the body to heal? There are so many different factors involved — it is individual to each of us. You would think that most food allergies would go away once you took sugar out of your diet — and that is true for some people but not true for everyone. Some people can just stop eating all sugar and after a few days or a few weeks their body bounces back to homeostasis and they feel much better. Other people need to do more than take sugar out of their diet. They need to find those foods to which they react and remove those from their diet also.

For some people it just takes a few weeks. Other people who were born with a genetically compromised endocrine system and then have abused their body for a long time will find that it takes a lot longer. For many of us, it is a lifetime practice.

⌒

3-DAY CARROT AND GREEN JUICE DIET

This 3-day juice fast or diet is a great way to kick off your new food regime. It helps to detoxify your liver and gallbladder while giving your digestive system and body a chance to rest.

During the fasting time, you might experience withdrawal symptoms such as headaches, fatigue, anger, perspiration, depression, and just general malaise. These symptoms usually do not last more than a week. When the withdrawal is over, you should feel much better because many of the toxins have left your body.

If you have a juicer and can juice the carrots and green vegetables fresh each day, I recommend that you do that. If you need to buy the juices, go to a health food store — and if they don't have the juices on hand, ask if they can order them for you. Make sure that the bought juices do not have fruit juice in them. Also buy one gallon of distilled water.

Every day for three days drink:

> 1 quart of green juice with
> 1 cup of carrot juice added, and
> *at least* 4 glasses of distilled water

For the green juices, you can use celery, lettuce, green peppers, cukes, spinach, or any other green vegetable that tastes good to you. You can drink these juices any way you want. You can sip the juices all day or drink one cup every two hours. You can have the juices over ice, or dilute them with water. If you want more than 4 glasses of water, drink it. You can have a litte lemon in your water if you like.

There are some fine herbal products that can be taken during a juice fast that help to detoxify. Look in your local health food store.

When you go back to Food Plan 3 after three days, your first meal should consist of just a few raw vegetables. For your second meal, eat just a few steamed vegetables. Your third meal might have a boiled egg and vegetables. By the second day of eating, you can eat any of the foods on Food Plan 3, unless you are testing individual foods for allergies.

THE HEALING FOOD PLANS

CAUTION: Following Food Plans 1, 2, or 3 may initiate withdrawal symptoms and a phenomenon called physiological and psychological detox. You may experience different symptoms, many similar to withdrawal from any addiction. Fever, depression, headaches, chills, anger, and fatigue are the most common symptoms. These will gradually lessen and then disappear, usually within a week to ten days.

Food Plan 1 — For maintaining health

This is the least restrictive food plan. If you generally feel well and have few symptoms, this is the plan for you.

1. Avoid all foods in Categories IV and V. Eat any other food.

2. If after being on this plan for seven days, you are not feeling better, your body chemistry requires a more comprehensive food plan. Therefore, proceed with Food Plan 2.

Food Plan 2 — For simple healing

This plan eliminates yeast, wheat, sugar, dairy, and citrus and restricts other fruits, nuts and seeds.

1. Avoid all foods in Categories III, IV, and V, and eat food in Category II only in small amounts and only between meals. For meals, eat Category I foods.

2. If after being on Plan 2 for seven days, you are still not experiencing better health, you need to proceed to Food Plan 3.

Food Plan 3 — For maximum healing

This is the healing plan; it focuses on fresh vegetables, beans and grains, and small portions of fish, meat, or poultry. Yeast, wheat, sugar, fruit, seeds and nuts, dairy, and caffeine are completely eliminated. It is clear that your unbalanced body chemistry involves more than just the common allergens.

Food Plan 3 is designed to provide complete nutrients to your body in their most bio-available form. Adherence to this plan automatically handles some complex food-related biochemical problems that Food Plans 1 and 2 did not handle. The procedures and foods of Food Plan 3 are the least stressful to your body chemistry.

1. For the next fourteen days eat only foods from Category I. Eat one small portion from each food group four or five times a day. Remember to follow the Ten Healthful Suggestions at the beginning of this chapter.

2. To maximize the healing effects of this food plan, you may want to start with the 3-day carrot and green juice fast described above.

3. If after fourteen days you are still not experiencing relief of symptoms, the problems you are having may be due to a medical problem. See a qualified practitioner who can give you blood tests and a test for food sensitivities to help you to find foods that do not upset your body chemistry.

Category III

Overcooking, overheating, and eating with sugar have turned these normally well-tolerated foods into potentially abusive foods. These foods can now unbalance the chemistry of those who have already impaired their ability to rebalance their body chemistry.

Yeast
Baker's yeast
Brewer's yeast
Mushrooms

Grains
Wheat bran
Wheat germ
White flour
Whole wheat flour

Fruits
Grapefruit
Mango
Orange
Tangerine

Herbs
Curry
Peppermint
Salt
Vanilla

Dairy
Blue cheese
Buttermilk
Cheese (all)
Cottage cheese
Cream cheese
Cow's milk
Whey
Yogurt

Nuts/Seeds
Cashew
Peanut

Miscellaneous
Cinnamon
Coffee
Coffee, decaf
Cola bean
Corn gluten
Cornstarch
Fructose
Honey
Hops
Molasses
Tea

Category II

If you have upset body chemistry, you may have become sensitive to these otherwise wholesome foods.

Fruits
Apple
Apricot
Avocado
Banana
Cantaloupe
Coconut
Cranberry
Fig
Grape
Guava
Melon (all)
Nectarine
Papaya
Peach
Pineapple
Plum (prune)
Raspberry
Strawberry
Watermelon

Nuts/Seeds
Almond
Brazil nut
Chestnut
Flax seed
Hazelnut
Hickory nut
Macadamia nut
Pecan
Pistachio
Safflower seed
Sunflower seed
Walnut

Herbs/Condiments
Allspice
Anise seed
Chicory
Clove
Cream of Tartar
Paprika
Spearmint

Category I

When prepared and eaten in a proper manner, these foods are the least stressful to your body chemistry. Remember that you individually may be allergic or sensitive to any food; all of the Food Plans need to be individually modified for each person.

Green Leafy Vegetables
Artichoke
Brussel sprouts
Cabbage
Kale
Lettuce (all)
Spinach

Green Vegetables
Alfalfa
Asparagus
Avocado
Broccoli
Celery
Chinese pea
Okra

Yellow/White Vegetables
Cauliflower
Corn
Cucumber
Squash (all)

Root Vegetables
Jicama
Onion
Parsnip
Potato
Radish
Rutabaga
Turnip

**Orange/Purple/
Red Vegetables**
Beet
Carrot
Eggplant
Pumpkin
Sweet potato
Tomato

Herbs/Condiments
Arrowroot
Basil
Bay leaf
Black pepper
Butter
Caraway

Herbs/Condiment Cont'd.
Carob
Chili pepper
Chive
Cilantro
Coconut
Dill
Garlic
Ginger
Horseradish
Lemon
Lime
Mustard
Nutmeg
Olive oil
Oregano
Parsley
Rose hip
Rosemary
Safflower oil
Sage
Sesame oil
Sunflower oil
Tarragon
Thyme

Fish
Anchovy
Bass
Catfish
Clam
Cod
Crab
Flounder
Haddock
Halibut
Mackerel
Oyster
Perch
Red Snapper
Salmon
Sardine
Scallop
Shark
Shrimp

Fish Cont'd.
Sole
Swordfish
Trout
Tuna
Any other fish

Meat/Poultry
Bacon
Beef
Chicken
Chicken egg
Duck
Frog's leg
Beef liver
Chicken liver
Lamb liver
Pheasant
Pork
Turkey
Venison

Beans/Grains
Azuki bean
Barley
Bean sprout
Kidney bean
Buckwheat
Garbanzo bean
Green pea
Black-eyed pea
Lentil
Lima bean
Millet
Navy bean
Oat
Pinto bean
Red bean
Brown rice
White rice
Wild rice
Rye
Soybean
Split pea
String bean
White bean

If you are a vegetarian, use our Food Plans, but eliminate the Meat group and combine beans and grains for complete protein.

Category IV

These foods are always abusive to human body chemistry. Only those who remain adaptive can rebalance their body chemistry after frequent exposure to Category IV foods. The more Category IV foods consumed, the more rapid the deterioration in the body chemistry.

Alcohol	Corn syrup
Beet sugar	Malt
Cane sugar	Maple sugar
Cocoa	Saccharin
Corn sugar	

Category V

These chemicals have known unbalancing effects on the body chemistry, and it serves your health to use them seldom and with caution.

Aspirin	MSG
Baking powder	Petroleum by-products
BHT	Sodium benzoate
Caffeine	Tobacco
Food coloring	Tylenol
Formaldehyde	

BUYING, STORING, AND PREPARING FOOD FOR HEALING

This is probably the most important section of this book, because it is all practical information about buying, preparing, cooking, and serving food. The rest of the book teaches you the theory, but if you can't put the theory into practice — if you don't know what you need to do in order to change what you put in your mouth — then all has been wasted.

Buying Food

Where can you buy fresh, healthy foods? Your choices are: supermarkets, health food stores, co-operatives, farmer's markets — or grow it yourself. It is, of course, ideal to grow the food yourself because you can control all the pesticides, fungicides, and chemical fertilizers that you use. This is not practical for most of us, but if you can, I certainly recommend it. The next best way as far as I'm concerned is to buy at a farmer's market where the farmers come to town every day, or once a week, or at a certain time, and bring fresh fruit and vegetables direct from the farms into the city. There's no middle man. The farmers are the ones who do the selling. I live in Santa Monica, California, and we have a farmer's market that comes once a week, every Wednesday afternoon. They set up their farm produce on a street in Santa Monica and we can all go down and buy off the back of trucks from various farmers. We can talk to each one of the farmers and determine whether their fruits and vegetables are organically grown or not. This way we get fresh vegetables and fruits without many of the fungicides, pesticides, dyes, and waxes we find in supermmarket produce. These foods are also fresher than most you buy elsewhere because they come straight from the farm.

I have noticed that some of these foods from farmers are not "picture perfect" in size and shape and therefore, many times they can't sell this produce to a market. On the other hand, those "perfect" tomatoes at the supermarket sure don't taste very good. I'd rather have smaller, larger, or imperfect shapes — and real flavor, freshness, and purity. Do check closely to see that the foods are not bruised or in any way not of high quality. Overall, I think you will be amazed at the price and the quality of the food that you get at these farmer's markets. And if you go on a trip and are in farming country, stop at a farm and get some fresh food.

The next best alternatives are health food stores and food co-ops. Most of the health food stores label whether their foods are from organic sources or not. Unfortunately, some of the foods have been shipped from long distances and their shelf life can be long. We get them after they have been shipped and stored and they're not as fresh as if you grew them yourself or brought them from a farmer.

If none of these options are available to you and you do buy your produce from a large chain grocery store, check the food carefully and when you get home be sure you scrub it thorough-ly. Some people are adding one teaspoon of Clorox™ bleach to one gallon of water in order to help eliminate the pesticides, fungicides, and sprays that are used during and after the farming process. I recommend that you shop at least twice a week because the less the food is stored, whether it be in a warehouse or a grocery store or at home, the more vitamins and minerals are retained and the foods are healthier and better for you.

By asking questions about the quality of our food, and by being concerned about what we put in our mouth, we can do fairly well in terms of eating healthy food. We can control which foods we put in our mouth, avoiding both abusive foods and foods we ourselves have abused.

Abusive foods are foods such as sugar, caffeine, rancid fats, hydrogenated fats, and over-heated foods. These are things everybody should avoid. Foods we have abused are those foods that we have eaten with sugar, that we have overcooked, or that we have eaten too much of. Our bodies have set up an allergic reaction to these foods.

The whole situation becomes more complicated when most of our foods are processed in some way. For instance, the fruits and vegetables at the supermarket were grown with chemical fertilizers, then during the growing process they are sprayed with pesticides, fungicides, and herbicides. Just before going to market many are sprayed again so that they will look garden-fresh when they get to your homes. Fruits and vegetables are not the only foods that have been tampered with. Our farm animals also eat food that have antibiotics and an alphabet soup of numerous other drugs in them. Chemicals such as growth hormones, antifungal sprays, pesticides, hormones, insecticides, herbicides, antibiotics, larvacides, tranquilizers, appetite stimulants, preservatives and coloring agents — and who knows what other unregulated and unauthorized drugs get into the food chain. There are between 20 and 30 thousand veterinary drugs and chemicals being used by agribusiness today. Of that startling number, a recent congressional subcommittee study revealed that 90% of those chemicals are being used illegally by agribusiness while the FDA looks the other way.

One example is diethylstilbestrol, known as DES, which was introduced into livestock production after W.W. II. It has since been banned by the federal government because it was discovered that DES caused cancer, even in the smallest doses imaginable. Yet today, many factory farms in the U.S. continue to use DES illegally. Others have changed to other sex hormones such as Steer-oid, Ralgro, Compudose, and Synovex which have very similar effects. Those hormones are used in virtually every food lot in the United States. Recently some large chain grocery stores have banned any meat with hormones. Let us hope that this trend will continue.

The living conditions of our farm animals are also an issue. These conditions are not only cruel to the animals but this cruelty puts such stress on their bodies that sickness and disease run rampant. Stress upsets their body chemistry, their mineral relationships, and compromises their immune system, just like it upsets human bodies. And they get diseases, just like we do. Because of the sickness, they need to take antibiotics. If they wouldn't keep chickens crammed in small cages and coops with four or five other chickens with an average of one square foot per chicken and keep them inside, stacked up in layers with artificial light, the chickens wouldn't need the antibiotics. At some chicken farms, up to 30% of the chickens die of disease before they are ready for the market. A U.S. Department of Agriculture agency has found that nearly 40% of all poultry leaves the slaughter plant contaminated with salmonella or other bacterial infections that could cause food poisoning. By comparison, the figure for beef and pork leaving the slaughter plants is less than 5 or 6% — it's hard to process 400 birds and keep the final product as clean as when processing a single steer or five hogs.

But beef and pork are also at risk. Most cows today are not range fed. Most are kept in stalls and are unable to exercise properly. To give you an idea of their living conditions, think of a 12 foot by 15 foot bedroom which is 180 square feet. Now put 13 half ton steers in that room. That is how they live.

And this is all about the so called "fresh" foods at your grocery store — the produce and meat. What about all the other sections in between? Almost all of the canned, boxed, and frozen foods in the aisles of your supermarket are filled with chemicals, unlabeled glucose, labeled sweeteners from corn syrup to dextrose to fructose to barley malt. Reading labels can be a frightening experience! My general rule is: If you don't recognize and can't pronounce the ingredients, don't buy the product.

So, what's the alternative? Truthfully, there are no easy answers. One must first maintain a detective posture anywhere food is sold today. That is absolutely imperative. Next, avoid supermarkets as much as possible and seek out smaller, independent health food retailers, wholesalers, and neighborhood co-ops. Be informed buyers, taking nothing for granted anymore. Ask plenty of questions. Beware of the new buzz words: "organic," "open range fed" and "all natural." One must be on guard since some health food store operators have been duped by clever advertising and ambiguous labeling which deceive the consumer into thinking they are buying a superior product.

Are Irradiated Foods the Answer?

A lot of the food we eat and our children eat may have first been irradiated by Cobalt 60 or Cesium 137. The proponents tell us such treatment is absolutely safe, that such irradiation can reduce the use of potentially dangerous pesticides, and that the longer shelf life of irradiated foods will help us to feed the poverty-stricken parts of the world.

Any way you look at irradiated food — texture, taste, amino acid analysis, electrophoresis, chromatography — it looks very different from raw, cooked, or canned food. Irradiation is definitely not just another process. The most important differences between irradiated and unirradiated food are the many invisible and potentially dangerous biochemical changes. New chemical species are found in the fats, in the proteins and amino acids, in the carbohydrates, and most likely in a number of the hormone precursors normally present in foods. This is the first time in the 4 million years of man's evolution that he has regularly ingested catalytically active amounts of these compounds, which are affectionately called URP's or "Unique Radiolytic Products." The "U" might well also stand for Unknown or Unidentified or Untested. Do you want yourself, your family, and your constituents to be unwitting guinea pigs in a long-term experiment? What an enormous liability!

Recent history has supplied us with a very long list of supposedly harmless compounds which have severely backfired, such as butter yellow, DES, thalidomide, asbestos, birth control pills, DDT, and EDB — and even antibiotics. Will URP's be next? No one can honestly say that they know. The very high energy of the irradiation produces many types of free radicals and also other unusual and highly reactive species which result in both volatile and non-volatile URP's, including the highly toxic benzene and other compounds never found in foods before. Their possible long-term cumulative effects include liver toxicity, allergic reactions, generalized changes in the immune system, carcinogenicity, and the potentiation of other carcinogens.

There has been some testing of irradiated food, but the results are unclear. Some tests concluded that irradiation caused no change in foods. Other tests indicated changes. For instance, one study concluded that prolonged feeding with irradiated meat and fish causes disturbances of protein and lipid metabolism, a decrease in body weight and a decrease in the number of offspring in experimental animals.

In another study it was shown that malnourished children fed irradiated wheat developed abnormal white blood cells in their body, while malnourished children fed non-irradiated wheat did not develop these abnormal cells.

Many people believe that the testing that is done is not sensitive enough to detect changes.

Fresh vegetables, fruits, and protein that have been irradiated have to be labeled. Unfortunately, food that has been irradiated and processed need not be labeled. All of us could be eating food that has been irradiated without knowing it. How unfortunate.

What all this means to us in terms of the body chemistry principal is that when food changes its chemical configuration we do not have the evolutionary enzymes to digest it; therefore these chemicals can get into the bloodstream and cause an immune response. The less immune responses we have the stronger our immune systems are to defend us against normal invaders such as bacteria, virus, and chemicals found in our society today.

I feel that there are still so many things that have not been tested on both a short term and long term basis with food irradiation that it would certainly be best for the consumer to avoid these foods.

Food Preparation

After you have brought the food home and washed it, I recommend that you keep it for storage in the refrigerator. Preparation of fresh food can be just as simple as fast foods, particularly if you are using a food slicer.

I am going to speak specifically about eating from Food Plan 3. These are foods that do not upset the body chemistry unless a person is allergic to one of them. As you can see, they consist of vegetables, small amounts of protein, beans and grains. Note that there are no wheat or dairy products on the chart. There are also no hydrogenated oils like margarine, no nuts, no seeds, and no fruits. Now these foods that I just mentioned are fine for a healthy person, but if you are not feeling well and your urine testing is not normal, these healthy foods could be upsetting your body chemistry. I'm going to address myself just to Food Plan 3 — the maximum healing plan — at the moment. You can modify if you are using Food Plan 1 or 2, because you will be eating all the food on Food Plan 3 anyway if you are on Food Plan 1 or 2. Notice the food has been divided into seven different food groups with different foods under each group. There are various reasons why I feel a person should eat small amounts out of each of the seven different groups.

I feel that every time you sit down to a meal, you should get all the fatty acids, all the amino acids, all the vitamins and minerals — 54 different nutrients. When you get all of these nutrients the body will have a better chance to absorb and assimilate the food and heal. So when a person eats a small amount from those seven different food groups, it is possible to get all of the 54 different nutrients. That is reason number one. Reason number two is that if you happen to be allergic to any one of those foods and you only have a small portion, only a small amount of undigested food will get into the bloodstream and will only cause small immune response and hopefully the body will still have the opportunity to heal itself.

Let's say you sit down and have a heaping bowl of pinto beans. Pinto beans are an evolutionary food, just like all the foods on this chart; nothing is wrong with some pinto beans with a small amount of butter. But if you sit down and eat a large bowl of them, and then realize that you are allergic to pinto beans, you would cause an immune response.

There's another reason why you don't want to sit down and eat a bowl of pinto beans. A person who has compromised his body due to abusive foods and an abusive lifestyle has enzymes which are not functioning as well as possible. If you eat more of one food than you have enzymes for, you exhaust the enzymes and then the food does not digest. Again it gets into the bloodstream undigested and again the immune system has to come into action. The reason for eating small amounts from a variety of foods is so that you will not exhaust your enzyme system because you will pull from a lot of enzyme systems in order to digest a variety of foods. In order to digest broccoli, you need five to six different enzymes, and a variety of minerals in small amounts. If you eat a small amount of beef, you will pull from some other enzyme systems. If you eat a small amount of carrots, you'll pull from still other enzyme systems. So, hopefully you won't exhaust your enzymes and that undigested food does not get into the bloodstream and cause havoc with your immune system.

Cooking

You may have to change some of your habits when you start "cooking for health," but a few simple guidelines should help you make the transition simply. First, as we discussed earlier, you should shop two or three times a week to make sure your food is fresh. You may need to think this through a little to find a way to fit the extra shopping into your schedule: think about before work and during your lunch hour, for instance. Next, you need to take 20 minutes or so when you get home to clean and store the food. Finally, you may want to invest in a food slicer and a steamer. From here on, though, your new way of eating and cooking should be very simple.

Breakfast tends to be a challenge on Food Plan 3: no muffins or Danish, no fried eggs or fried potatoes — oh dear, what else is there? Well, how about veggies and rice? You could slice up many of the different foods from the food groups and pop them into a stainless steel steamer and steam them over a small amount of water. When you slice them thin, you will find it will take only 5 minutes to cook. You could put all of those vegetable into a steamer, you could put fish, chicken sliced thin, beef sliced thin, or ground beef into the steamer — you could cook them all at once. The only two things that you need to precook are the rice and beans. You could cook more beans or rice than needed for one meal, and freeze this food. Then thaw it and steam it with other fresh vegetables. Also you can cook double or triple the amount you need for your breakfast. At breakfast time you can eat the veggies with a small amount of butter and eat them hot. Then you can take some more of the vegetables and put a mayonnaise or salad dressing on them and have them for lunch.

Veggies for breakfast too radical an idea for you? Let me give you some other suggestions. Health food stores carry barley, quinoa, or rice cereals which you might cook and eat with butter. But remember Food Plan 3 is small amounts from a variety of foods so don't eat too much of any cereal. With the cereal, you might have one boiled egg, a rice cracker, sliced tomatoes, and steamed potatoes. Another idea is to take a rice cracker and add sliced avocado, sliced onions and sliced tomato, or a corn tortilla with a poached egg over it and some tomato salsa; throw in a little guacamole, tomatoes, and lettuce if that sounds good to you.

SIMPLE SUGGESTIONS FOR BREAKFASTS AND SNACKS

1. Bake potatoes the night before and refrigerate. In the morning slice the potatoes and saute in butter at a low temperature.

2. Baked potato with butter, guacamole, or pureed beans.

3. Corn tortilla with butter, tomatoes, an egg, and/or guacamole.

4. Oatmeal with butter.

5. Cream of Rice with butter.

6. Rice cakes with sliced avocado, tomato, onion, green pepper, or cucumber.

7. One-egg omelet with sliced tomatoes, cut-up potatoes, green pepper, onion, or other vegetables.

8. One-egg ranchero with corn tortilla.

9. Cooked rice with butter.

10. Steamed sweet potato with butter. Sweet potatoes are also good cold. They taste like candy.

11. One cup of popped corn.

12. My favorite quick breakfast is leftover rice heated with grated carrots, frozen peas, frozen lima beans, and butter.

At lunch you could use the same vegetables that you cooked for breakfast but cooled with a salad dressing on them. If you go out for lunch, you could have a salad or some fish and a baked potato, or some rice. For dinner you might have a soup or a stew, checking to make sure you are not allergic to any of the ingredients. Many of the recipes that you have used in the past for stews or soups can still be used. Just eliminate any sugar, substitute arrowroot for wheat as a thickener and eliminate any foods to which you react. Don't use milk for a soup base. You might use vegetable or chicken stock, or a can of tomato or V-8 Juice as a base.

I keep a plastic bag in my refrigerator that has six or seven different vegetables in it and then I just pull the plastic bag out, slice the vegetables with a slicer and drop them in my steamer.

The more raw food you can eat the better. Raw food has many more enzymes and the food has not been depleted of its nutrients through the heating process. But some sick people cannot handle raw food — it gives them diarrhea, cramps, or bloating. If this happens to you with raw food, just steam your vegetables lightly and eat them with small amounts of protein for a few weeks and then try some raw vegetables again. At the beginning just eat a few raw vegetables at a time, then slowly add more as your body can handle the raw foods.

Remember not to overcook your food because it is much more difficult to digest. Every food is made of four elements: nitrogen, carbon, oxygen and hydrogen in different chemical configurations. Broccoli will have one chemical configuration and beef another. We have evolutionary enzymes to digest those foods in their chemical configurations. Each food also has its own heat labile point. It is that point where food changes its chemical configuration, when we heat it to too high a temperature. When this happens, we do not have the enzymes to digest the food and therefore it can putrefy in the gut, get into the bloodstream undigested and cause an immune response. So if you burn your toast, throw it out; better wasted outside than inside.

Let me talk a minute about eating at a restaurant. When eating in restaurants, the only place I have a hard time is in a pizza parlor; other than that I can find pretty much what I want. At a fish restaurant, a French restaurant, Italian or most any other restaurants, they serve protein in the form of fish, meat, and poultry. Many times the restaurant serves too much protein — people are advertising half-pounders, quarter-pounders, a pound of lobster — that's too much protein. So, eat part of it and take the rest home for tomorrow. You can usually get a potato or rice and some vegetables and a salad. You really can eat a meal in a restaurant that has all of the nutrients that you need. If you don't get something from all the seven food groups, there's no reason to worry. When you eat out, just do the best you can and enjoy yourself. It might be a good idea to bless the food and then it will even be easier on the body. Some people hold hands before dinner or say a prayer. Whatever fits your beliefs, take a moment to relax and to be grateful before taking your food.

Breakfast is difficult to eat out, I have a hard time with it. Let me give you a couple of suggestions. If you are able to eat fruit alone without having any reaction, you might just have fruit for breakfast, nothing else. Be careful, don't order canned fruit. It is usually filled with a syrup that has sugar in it. Try to get whole fresh fruit, not juice. Here is another suggestion. Restaurants usually have some form of hot cereals, such as oatmeal or cream of wheat — but remember not to eat a large portion. A third suggestion might be to ask the restaurant to poach or boil one egg and hope that they have some fresh potatoes, not the dehydrated or canned type, but some fresh potatoes that they saute lightly. So you could have potatoes and ask them possibly for some sliced tomatoes if you are not eating bread or wheat. These are a couple of ideas for breakfast in a restaurant, but yes, it is hard, the hardest meal to eat out.

CAN A VEGETARIAN USE THE FOOD PLANS?

If you are a vegetarian, our program will suit you very well. On any one of the food plans you will be able to combine beans and grains to get complete protein. Many meat eaters in our society are "protein-logged" today — bacon and eggs for breakfast, hamburgers for lunch, and meat and potatoes for dinner. That is too much protein. There is research to show that when a person eats an excess amount of protein at one meal, calcium is excreted in the urine which can lead to osteoporosis and other diseases. Unfortunately, it is not only the amount of protein that you eat but the way you cook it that is the problem. If you fry the bacon and eggs for breakfast, you overheat the food. When you overcook anything, it will pass the heat labile point and change its chemical configuration. The fat and protein can get into the bloodstream undigested and cause problems. The undigested fat can clog the arteries and cause heart disease and then the undigested protein and fat can become a food allergy. Of course, undigested food not only can clog the arteries but also may cause other problems such as psoriasis, arthritis or headaches. If you are a vegetarian you do not have any of these problems because you do not eat any of those foods.

However, you may still be eating sugar. Since the body manufactures its own cholesterol even if you do not eat it, eating sugar can clog the arteries if your genetic blueprint is to get heart disease and you upset your body chemistry. Many vegetarians have eliminated sugar which certainly is a good idea.

If you are not a vegetarian you do not have to have these problems either, but chances are that you might because of the ways meats and fats are cooked in our restaurants. A meat eater should remember to boil, poach, steam or bake chicken, fish, meat or eggs rather than fry, saute or barbecue, and remember to eat small portions.

Because a vegetarian needs the same amount of calories that a meat eater does, he needs to consume more vegetables and grains, which do not have as high a concentration of calories per ounce as meat or fish.

There are many books on vegetarianism. I recommend that if you are a vegetarian you read on. A person who chooses to eat no eggs or milk products needs to have a clear picture of protein and how we assimilate it. This is not a problem, it just needs to be studied.

A study from a highly regarded professor at Yale compared the stamina and strength of meat eaters against those of vegetarians. Professor Irving Fisher selected men from three groups: meat-eating athletes, vegetarian athletes, and vegetarian sedentary subjects. Fisher reported the results of his study in the Yale Medical Journal. He found that the flesh eaters showed far less endurance than the vegetarians, even when the latter led a sedentary life. Fisher concluded that the difference in endurance between the flesh eaters and the vegetarians was due entirely to the difference in their diet. There is strong evidence that a non-flesh diet is conductive to endurance. Whenever similar tests have been done, the results have been similar. This does not lend a lot of support to the supposed association of meat with strength and stamina.

Remember, there are a variety of ways to eat well and allow your body to heal. In Chapter 5, we will look more closely at factors such as emotion and lifestyle and how they relate to our digestion, our body chemistry, and our immune system.

CHAPTER 5

Toward a Healing Lifestyle: The Four Arenas

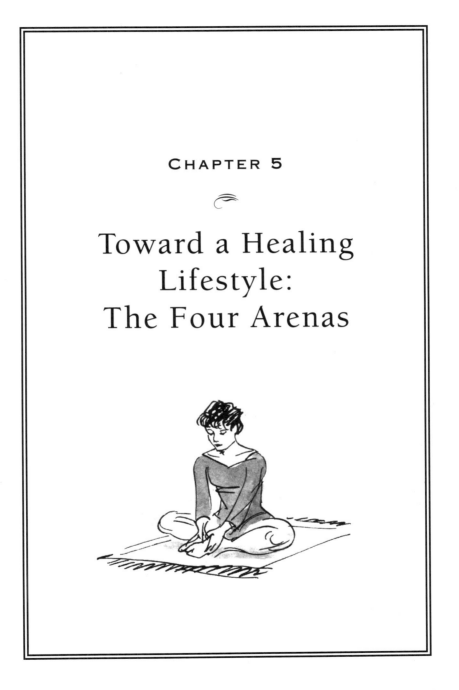

The Four Arenas

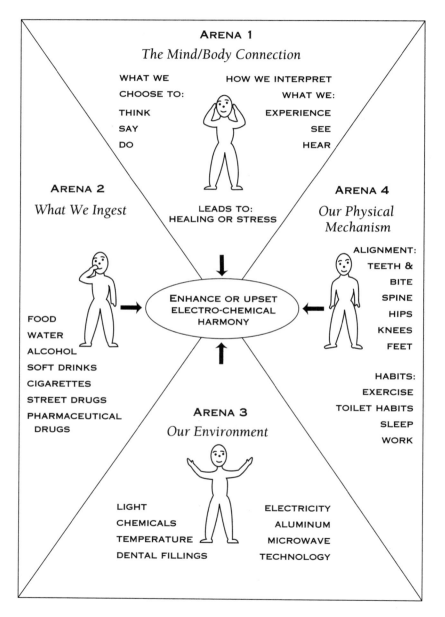

ARENA 1

The Mind/Body Connection

WHAT WE
CHOOSE TO:

THINK
SAY
DO

HOW WE INTERPRET
WHAT WE:

EXPERIENCE
SEE
HEAR

LEADS TO:
HEALING OR STRESS

ARENA 2

What We Ingest

FOOD
WATER
ALCOHOL
SOFT DRINKS
CIGARETTES
STREET DRUGS
PHARMACEUTICAL
 DRUGS

ENHANCE OR UPSET
ELECTRO-CHEMICAL
HARMONY

ARENA 4

*Our Physical
Mechanism*

ALIGNMENT:
TEETH &
BITE
SPINE
HIPS
KNEES
FEET

HABITS:
EXERCISE
TOILET HABITS
SLEEP
WORK

ARENA 3

Our Environment

LIGHT
CHEMICALS
TEMPERATURE
DENTAL FILLINGS

ELECTRICITY
ALUMINUM
MICROWAVE
TECHNOLOGY

In the previous chapters you have read that our 20th century lifestyle can upset our body chemistry and take us out of homeostasis. This chapter will break that lifestyle into four arenas of activity and talk about how we can positively influence those arenas. We will talk about four arenas in which our actions produce basic effects on our electrochemical balance. When we upset our bodies, we upset this delicate balance and then the minerals change relationships, the enzymes cannot function as well, all of food does not digest, undigested food gets into the bloodstream, and an immune response is triggered. This is the problem — the secret to natural healing is learning how to get your body into balance and keep it there. Practically, this means keeping your system strong and your immune defenses undepleted — so that even when the unavoidable challenges of 20th century living throw us out of homeostasis, our bodies can bounce back quickly, and stay balanced longer.

ARENA 1: THE MIND-BODY CONNECTION

Doctors are rethinking medicine's time-honored tenet that the mind and body are distinct and separate entities. More and more we are realizing that there is a strong mind-body connection.

Many times our head gets in the way of our body getting well. Our body is just a stimulus/response mechanism. It can only respond to what happens to it. Responses are not right or wrong or good or bad — they are just the only response the machine is geared to give. If you are angry when you eat, certain chemicals are released, certain electrical signals are triggered — your body responds in its pre-arranged way. If you are happy when you eat, your body will respond in another way.

Let's look at an example. If someone is angry and yells at you, you have some choices about how you will react: You can take it personally. You can internalize it. You can get angry back. But none of these responses will enhance your body's natural healing mode. The best way to deal with this situation is to decide that this is not your problem; it is the other person's problem — it is the other person's anger. Of course, it is difficult when someone comes to you in anger. It is a put-off. But really, anger is rarely the real issue; anger almost always covers up pain. So rather than get angry, try to find what the pain is and deal with that pain. And remember this when you are angry, too: it is also easier for the other person to hear your pain than your anger. The person is more likely to be sensitive.

If you do become distressed by anger, depression, rage, or holding judgments against others, then I suggest that you do not eat or eat very simply, because it will be difficult for that food to digest. Instead, go exercise, run, take a deep breath, have a bubble bath, listen to a relaxation tape, meditate, pray — do something to take the stress off your body. To paraphrase Mark Braunstein, "The person who eats beer and franks with cheer and thanks will probably be healthier than the person who eats sprouts and bread with doubts and dread."

Need more ideas? Here are some more things you can do to reduce stress that do not include quitting your job or divorcing your spouse. Read a book. Books abound on this subject. Or just read for pleasure, about any topic. Take some time for yourself. Listen to a relaxation tape, or learn about some aspect of self-help. There are many cassette tapes available today and you can listen at home or in your car as you commute to work. Check with your local library and bookstores, too: many libraries, bookstores, and music stores have a list of available tapes just for the asking. Go to a workshop. Most cities have weekend workshops that can be attended by anyone for a fee. These can be the start of understanding why you are stressed. Remember there are also good counselors around — and don't be intimated about "shopping around" until you find someone you can relate to with ease.

It is possible, as Norman Cousins suggests in his book, *An Anatomy of an Illness*, to harness the healing powers of the mind. Studies show that life's stresses, such as the death of a spouse, loss of a job, or severe depression can impair immune system function. We all have stressful events in our lives. The way a person handles stressful events is more important in determining whether one suffers ill effects than the event itself.

There is interesting research to show exactly what stress can do to a body. One researcher found no difference between the number of stressful events (such as marriage problems, death) in a study done of heavy smokers. However, what this research found was that those smokers who developed lung cancer perceived these events as being more negative and felt more guilty about them than did those who did not develop the cancer.

In another study researchers found that certain neurotransmitters, which are the messengers that allow nerve cells to communicate with one another, can suppress the killer T-cells that are part of our immune system and attack foreign invaders. When one of these T-cells attacks an invader, receptors appear on the invader's surface. Neurotransmitters fit into these receptors much as a key fits into a lock. Acetylcholine is one of these neurotransmitters, and it enhances the ability of the T-cells to do their job. But other neurotransmitters, like epinephrine (adrenaline) and dopamine, impair the killing capacity of the T-cells and suppress the immune system. And these other neurotransmitters are the ones that are released in response to stress. So the more stressed you are, the more suppressed your immune system is likely to be. And we all know this from our own experience: when we are tired and run down, we are much more likely to get sick — it is part of the "when it rains, it pours" syndrome.

Qualities of the Self-Healing Person

Why is it that some people rarely get sick and when they do, they get well rapidly? I think that we can learn from these people. Here are a few of the things that they have in common.

Self-healing people view life as a challenge rather than as threat. These people live life to the fullest. Self-healers seem to share a feeling of control. There are two types of quick recoverers. The first type are extroverts who seek out stimulation, are spontaneous and fun-loving. The second type are active and involved, but also calm and bemused. These people choose to have only a few close friends, although they also enjoy the presence of others. The self-healing personality has an exuberance which affects others. The core of good health of these people is positive emotions, a sense of choice in one's life, and a sense of creative self-fulfillment.

If you have ever been called eccentric, you will like the following information. According to a psychologist in Scotland, being eccentric may help you live a longer-than-average life. 300 Britons and 800 Americans who are described, and sometimes describe themselves, as being eccentric (including a farmer who sometimes lectures his sheep on the dangers of conformity and a woman who has 1000 plastic gnomes in her garden) were asked about their general health, behavior, and lifestyle. As a group, eccentrics tend to be loners, have strong senses of humor, are very intelligent, and are often preoccupied with one subject. These eccentrics feel ill enough to visit a doctor on average only once every 8 years compared to about 3 times a year for the population at large. They are mentally fit, tend to describe themselves as happy and since they don't feel the need to conform to societal rules, are relatively free of stress. Based on current data and a review of some 400 eccentrics throughout modern history, overall eccentrics live five to ten years longer than average. So the next time you feel like doing something just a little bit odd — go ahead and do it!

As far as I'm concerned, life is very exciting. There are so many things that I want to do in life. I want to see the world — every corner. I want to tell people what I know about health because it is very painful for me to see people go through life in physical or mental pain when I know that it is not necessary. I have at least 18 books I want to read. Some day I am going to learn how to do off-loom weaving. I'd like to take a class in cultural geography. My list goes on — I hope that you are also excited about the possibilities out there. They are endless.

ARENA 2: WHAT WE INGEST

In addition to the concerns we have been talking about all along in terms of abusive foods like sugar and alcohol and foods that we have abused through overeating or eating in combination with abusive foods or stress, there are several other categories of "ingestibles" that deserve attention.

Food and Sickness: I don't believe in the old saying, "Feed a cold and starve a fever." I say you should starve a cold and starve a fever — with any kind of sickness, you have an upset body chemistry, a body out of homeostasis. At those times, it is better not to eat very much food. Just eat a minimum of food because your minerals will be upset and your enzymes will not be able to function as well. You might just drink broths or puree your food. Eat small amounts during the day but drink lots of water. Never eat large amounts — and chew, chew, chew. If you drink fruit juices, drink small amounts, perferably watered down, and drink them alone. Any food you eat is not going to digest as well, and you may become allergic to that food. When you are sick and you eat, you could get abdominal symptoms or any other symptoms. Consider food rotation: try not to eat the same food more than once every two or three days. You also might try some digestive enzymes. Remember that this upset is only temporary. When you regain your health you will find that the food that upset your stomach while you were sick no longer does that. When your body is balanced, the food will digest again. Don't forget to chew your food thoroughly. Digestion begins in the mouth.

Also remember that sickness puts stress on your body. At this time, you need more rest. So slow down, sleep more, and give your body a chance to rest and heal.

Water: Make sure you drink enough water to stay hydrated — and drink most of it between meals. The old rule of thumb of six to eight 8-oz glasses of water a day is a good one. And remember — this is in addition to any other liquids you are taking. Unfortunately, many of our water systems are polluted. Filtered water or bottled water might be a good idea in many areas of the United States. And do a little research on the kind of bottled water you buy — some of them have just as many contaminants as local tap water. It is my opinion that the safest alternative is a high-quality water filter system that you attach to your sink — and maintain by changing the filter often.

Alcohol: Alcohol is a simple sugar. It takes the same path through the body that sugar does. It can reach the blood stream from right under the tongue and never go through the digestive tract. There is enough research concerning alcohol to show that it robs the bones of calcium, upsets the body chemistry, can do damage to the liver, and is addictive. It is the number one abusive substance in the United States.

Soft drinks: I do not think that soft drinks should be taken by anyone even if they are sugar and caffeine free. All soft drinks have phosphoric acid in them. Phosphoric acid makes them bubble but also upsets the calcium/phosphorus ratio and makes you secrete excess calcium into your urine. This can deplete calcium from your bones, upset your body chemistry, and suppress your immune system. Sparkling lemon water is a good substitute — read the label to make sure it does not contain phosphoric acid or excess sodium.

Smoking: Enough has been said about smoking. Even the Surgeon General has had his say — you know you shouldn't smoke. But even nonsmokers are at risk; the effects of "secondhand smoke" are just beginning to be studied and documented. Researchers have discovered that secondhand smoke reduces the nonsmoker's ability to exercise effectively, for instance. Carbon monoxide, a colorless, odorless gas found in cigarette smoke, hampers the transportation of oxygen by red blood cells. In addition, evidence suggests that secondhand smoke makes your blood platelets abnormally sticky and more likely to clump together and form clots. These clots can stick to the coronary artery walls (among other places). The researchers concluded that nonsmokers who live with smokers increase their risk of heart disease and heart attack about 30% compared to nonsmokers who live and work in nonsmoking environments.

Drugs, pharmaceutical: I subscribe to many medical journals and newspapers. Each issue seems to tell of another drug that the FDA has taken off the market because of the longterm ill effects. I don't have time to talk about all of these drugs, but I would like to say a few words about antibiotics. Antibiotics have saved many lives and they definitely have a place in healing today. Unfortunately, they have also been grossly overused and do have serious side effects. The immune system becomes depressed. The phagocytes — the part of our immune system that gobbles up foreign invaders — do not function as well. As a result, after being on antibiotics for ten days, your body's natural healing capacity is supressed, and you are actually more susceptible to disease than before taking the drugs. Another problem is the overgrowth of a yeast called *Candida albicans* in the presence of antibiotics in the body. There is a section on treating *Candida* through diet modification in Chapter 6: Healing for Specific Conditions.

I read in The Johns Hopkins Medical Letter that 125,000 Americans die each year as a result of their pharmaceutical prescriptions. In 1989, the General Accounting Office released findings indicating that 51.5% of all drugs approved from 1976 to 1985 by the Federal Drug Administration (the FDA) carried "serious post-approval risk." The report revealed a virtually non-existent post-approval drug review procedure. My recommendation is to take as few pharmaceutical drugs as possible, and only under the direct supervision of a physician. Rather than taking the drugs, find out what you are doing that is causing the need to take drugs — and stop doing it!

ARENA 3: OUR ENVIRONMENT

Our surroundings play a large role in our body chemistry. Each day we make choices as to what we will do that can enhance or upset our body chemistry.

Light: Light plays an important part in our mental health. If you live in an area of the country where the sun doesn't shine for weeks at a time in the winter, I suggest that you do a little light therapy, especially if you get the winter blahs or some form of depression. This condition is now recognized as SAD: Seasonal Affect Disorder. Luckily, the solution is very simple: Light therapy involves simply sitting in front of a bright, full-spectrum light for a certain period of time each day. You might try 10 minutes to start and increase to 20 minutes if needed.

Temperature: Too much heat (*hyper*thermia) or too much cold (*hypo*thermia) can be a problem. If you get overheated, cooling off in a tepid bath can slowly and surely bring your temperature down. When you are overexposed to cold, taking a warm bath can elevate your temperature, as well as drinking a warm drink and using blankets that have been heated. Make sure you heat the body as well as the limbs. Your mother was really on to something when she told you to stay warm and dry: getting a chill can suppress your immune system and leave you more susceptible to a cold or infection.

Dental Fillings: For some people, the mercury in amalgam ("silver") fillings may play a role in diseases of the mouth as well as health problems in general. In one study a group of people with amalgam fillings exhibited a 250% greater frequency of oral health problems than did the non-amalgam group. Some of these problems were foul breath, bleeding gums, grinding teeth, metallic taste, and periodontal disease. Before you decide to have your amalgam fillings replaced, however, I recommend that you put your body back in homeostasis and let it heal. There are people who have amalgam fillings who have no symptoms and there are also people who have their fillings replaced and still have symptoms. So first of all, balance your body chemistry — and many symptoms will go away.

Technology: Technology is a double edged sword — don't abuse it. Televisions emit low grade ionized radiation — sit at least 10 feet away while watching TV.

Microwave cooking does the same thing — and in addition it seems to change the molecular structure of the food. When the molecular structure of food is changed, it is more difficult to digest because we do not have enzymes to digest food that has been re-structured. I suggest that you use other forms of cooking, although I do sometimes use a microwave oven to reheat food or heat water, but not to cook. If you *do* use microwaves for heating, be sure you do not stand in front of it when it is in use.

To minimize possible dangerous exposure to electromagnetic fields, stay several feet away from appliances that produce such fields. The recommended distance for fans is 2-3 feet, for electric clocks and alarm clocks: 3-4 feet, computers: 3-4 feet, copying machines, laser printers, and fax machines: 5 feet. Electric blankets also produce an electric field which may increase the risk of breast cancer. Turn on your electric blanket before you retire, but turn it off before you get into bed — then you will be toasty without getting toasted!

I feel strongly that aluminum cookware has no place in any kitchen. Research shows that when water in aluminum cookware is heated to only 88 degrees (water boils at 212 degrees), there is a 74-fold increase in aluminum in the water. That is more than 30 times the recommended water quality limit. There is some evidence that links excess aluminum with Alzheimer's disease and other conditions.

If you work all day long in a space that has fluorescent lighting, you might think of replacing those flourescent bulbs with full spectrum bulbs. These are available at many health food stores and often at hardware stores as well. They fit into the same light fixture, but are much kinder to the body. They can help with SAD as well (Seasonal Affect Disorder).

If you are sensitive to chemicals, do not paint your house until you have looked into mercury-free or non-toxic paints. Some brands of interior water-based latex paints, especially those produced before Aug 1990, contain mercury that can be inhaled through the lungs and accumulate in the body. The EPA (Environmental Protection Agency) announced that mercury could no longer be added to paints after Aug 20, 1990. I suggest you use paints that have been manufactured after that date. There are also special non-toxic paints available by mail order. These paints are a little more trouble to get and to apply, but for people suffering from chemical sensitivities, they can be well worth it.

New carpets cause problems for a lot of people; they can "outgas" for a long time — weeks or even months. If you redecorate, you might paint and recarpet and then take a long weekend or vacation away from your home to give the paint and carpet a chance to discharge their chemical-filled fumes. Leave as many windows open as possible. And even after you come back, leave the windows open as much as possible for several weeks.

Use as few chemicals in your home as possible. Today there are many alternatives, and besides health food stores, catalogs abound with natural products. Dry clean only those garments that absolutely can't be laundered — most wool and silk can be hand washed in special soaps with cool water. The most commonly used dry-cleaning chemical, perchloroethylene (PCE), has many problems. It pollutes water, may damage the ozone layer, and may cause cancer. And protect the ozone layer by refraining from using sprays to freshen your surroundings or to kill unwanted insects.

Several clinics in California specialize in treating patients who have been exposed to toxic substances, including chemical industry workers, Vietnam veterans who were exposed to Agent Orange, and several hundred other patients a year who suffer the ill effects of contact with the 55,000 man-made chemicals that are now in commercial production around the world. Their patients alternate daily sessions of moderate exercise and sauna treatments to clear out the chemicals that build up in the tissues that can cause headaches, fatigue, muscle aches, confusion, and skin disorders as long as twenty years after exposure. Patients also take gradually increasing doses of niacin to help flush toxins from tissues into the bloodstream, polyunsaturated oils to cleanse the intestines of chemicals, and mineral/vitamin supplements to replace nutrients that have been lost through sweat. This type of treatment is not necessary for average exposure to chemicals, but I recommend that you keep your exposure down to as little as possible, and think in terms of "detox" for yourself — regularly exercise and work up a sweat, drink plenty of fluids and help your system clear itself out.

Research shows that classical and new age music enhances body chemistry and hard rock upsets body chemistry. Remember those old studies with plants that were done in the sixties — and your parents clipped for you so you'd stop listening to "that awful noise"? Well, again, it seems that Mom and Dad were on to something: at least while you eat, there is evidence to favor slow melodic music. It not only helps in digestion but research shows that it also helps you eat less — while fast music makes you eat more.

ARENA 4: MAINTAINING THE PHYSICAL MACHINE

A body out of alignment, whether jaws, cranium, spine, hips or feet, will experience distress. Distress, in turn, upsets mineral relationships. Putting the body into alignment is easy to deal with if the other three arenas are in balance. A chiropractor makes an adjustment, and it will hold — because there is good protein digestion and tissue integrity. If you find you have to keep repeating the same chiropractic adjustment, consider the whole: is your body chemistry out of balance? If you are not functioning well in other areas, and mineral relationships have been upset, tissue integrity will be compromised. The four arenas are interrelated; each must be balanced before health is achieved.

Exercise: I must emphasize how important exercise is for the body. I speak of it later (Chapter 6) in terms of osteoporosis, but exercise is vital for everyone — whether or not osteoporosis is an issue. Exercise helps to balance the body chemistry — especially exercise that balances and centers, such as yoga, walking, running, tennis, or aerobics. New research shows there is a direct link between exercise and normal blood glucose. So even if you find you can't do any exercise, remember to breathe deeply 8 or 10 times every day.

Proper practice of yoga-type exercise can affect structure as well. Proper posture and alignment are very important components of health and fitness. When your spine is strong and flexible, proper alignment naturally follows. When your skeletal support is properly aligned, your weight is evenly distributed and your physical structure is balanced. And when you start your exercise from this kind of balance, injury is much less likely, recovery is fast, and the effort of your exercise is properly and evenly distributed. Balance is easier to maintain.

As we get older, it becomes more and more important to stretch and exercise. I think it takes longer for our body to respond as we age but if we continue to stretch and exercise all of our life, our body will respond easier as we age. I feel that a woman can start exercising at any time in her life, even if she has not done exercise before. Every community has classes in low impact aerobics, stretch, and yoga. Rudra Press has audio and video tapes you can use at home. Start today: take a brisk walk, swinging your arms, and taking deep, full breaths.

Dr. Kenneth Cooper, a leader in exercise research and promotion, found a direct link between premature death and poor physical fitness. Researchers found that in a study of over 13,000 men and women who attended his center between 1970 and 1985, men in the bottom 20% of fitness rankings were twice as likely to die early as their most fit counterparts. The early death rate of the least fit women in the study was four times that of those in the best shape.

Cooper's research suggests that regular exercise not only reduces the risk of death by heart attack — an already documented link — but even lowers the chances of dying from other chronic diseases, including cancer. What's more, for those in the fitness category just above the lowest level, the researchers discovered that the risk of premature death was significantly lower than for the least fit. That means that even modest exercise — like 30 minutes of brisk walking a day — might add years of life for people who have been totally inactive.

Light to moderate exercise seems to enhance the immune system, making us less susceptible to disease. But here, as in most things, the phrase "nothing in excess" is also true. While it will not be an issue for most of us, research has shown that prolonged, exhausting exercise can actually depress the immune system for a short period of time. Nordic skiers were tested for their salivary antibody (IgA) level after a 50 kilometer competition for men and a 20 kilometer run for women. Depressed IgA levels made the skiers far more susceptible to upper respiratory infections. This led to findings that various depleting physical activities cause immune efficiency to drop. Regular, moderate exercise is the key to balance.

I think you will find this research from the Human Performance Laboratory at Montana State University interesting, because athletes have generally accepted the axiom that a sugary snack before competition will boost your body's energy level. Scientists now know that while sugar does momentarily raise the blood sugar level, the response of insulin quickly drives it back down — often to below the pre-snack level. A recent test conducted at the Human Performance Laboratory confirmed that performance actually suffers after ingestion of sugar. Five distance runners were given a sugared drink and then asked to ride a stationary bicycle to the point of exhaustion. Three days later, the test was repeated, only this time they were given a sugar-free, caffeine-free cola. Exercise time to exhaustion was 25% longer after consuming the sugar-free drink. The message here is to avoid sugar, *not* that we should all drink sugar-free softdrinks! And if you are looking for calories, what you want is the complex carbohydrates, not the simple sugars. Good things to eat include whole wheat bread, crackers, potatoes, rice, beans and nuts.

Here's a partial list of medical problems that are helped by exercise:

- Osteoporosis — exercise helps to keep the bones strong. Mechanical stress acting on the bones results in increased mineralization of the bone.

- Obesity — not only do you work off calories during exercise, but you also increase the metabolic rate so that after exercise you continue to work off more calories.

- Cardiovascular function — exercise helps to speed up the blood in the blood vessels and also helps to clear the vessels.

- Stress reduction — exercise helps increase the metabolic functions in the body.

- Osteoarthritis — exercise of your hips, legs, shoulders, and arms prevents calcium deposits and will break up deposits that are already forming.

- Diabetes — adult onset diabetes is less likely to develop in active than in inactive people. Once diabetes has developed, regular exercise may increase insulin sensitivity which helps in the long term control of the disease and its complications.

- Hypertension — less likely to develop in those who exercise than in those who do not. Research shows that exercise

can bring down diastolic pressure from 5 to 25 mm Hg
and systolic pressure down by 3 to 15 mm Hg for those
who have high blood pressure.

- Cancer — studies of women college athletes showed that
  they had an 86% lower lifetime risk of breast cancer and
  a 162% lower lifetime risk of uterine cancer than non-
  athletic classmates.

There is no doubt. Exercise is important to everyone. I suggest
that you find some sport or activity that you enjoy (even dancing
will do) and do it 3 or 4 times a week. I love to play tennis and
also like to climb stairs which I do every day. I try to stretch once
a week and probably twice a week would be better. I get a high
after I exercise — I can feel my whole body hum.

Overwork: I love life, I find my work stimulating, and I work
long hours. No matter how much you love your work, though,
you can overwork and distress your body. Let me give you a
recent example: I was invited to Redding, California to lecture.
Over a three day period I gave lectures to five different groups
and counselled some clients individually. I was eating very well
and seemed to be getting enough sleep. But by the time I left
that city, I was exhausted and had a fierce headache. Even
though I loved what I was doing (stress is not only related to
things you hate . . . .) I didn't get enough rest and play time. The
body can't take too much of that kind of distress without symptoms occurring. Make sure that you take the time for rest and
relaxation, even if you do love your work. You might add to the
saying: "All work and no play make Jack a dull boy": "And it
may make him a dead boy."

Sleep: It is a good idea to have a minimum of six hours and a maximum of eight hours of sleep each night. Make sure you keep warm in the daytime and sleep warm at night.

Toilet Habits: When nature calls, you should answer — or nature may stop calling! Our body wants to get rid of its waste products. If you make a habit of "holding it" you force the body to take endols, cadaverines, and other putrefaction by-products back into your system. Then the immune system has to deal with it. If you are already compromising your immune system, it can become exhausted.

Some of us take better care of our cars or our pets than of ourselves. I hope the many suggestions for taking charge of your own health and activitating your body's natural healing mode in this book will encourage you to keep up with your pets and cars!

CHAPTER 6

Healing for
Specific Conditions

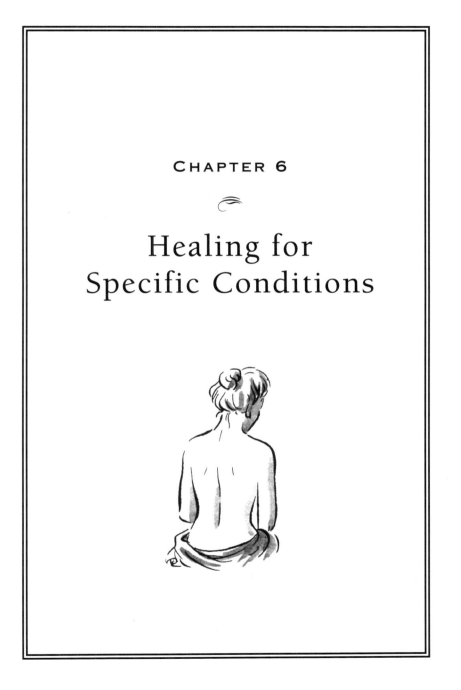

Healing for Specific Conditions

- OVERWEIGHT AND OBESITY

- OSTEOPOROSIS

- ARTHRITIS AND "TOXIC" CALCIUM

- HYPOTHYROIDISM

- HYPOGLYCEMIA AND DIABETES

- CANDIDA ALBICANS

- THE UNIVERSAL REACTOR: SEVERE ENVIRONMENTAL SENSITIVITY

- THE SPECIAL HEALTH NEEDS OF WOMEN

  - PMS
  - MENOPAUSE
  - THE BIRTH CONTROL PILL

Starting a diet is like starting a love affair. In the beginning, we live in a fantasy — everything seems wonderful, but we are afraid to ask the questions for fear of the answers. Many times we do not deal with the facts. Our fantasies often have little to do with reality. And when reality finally arrives, it can be very painful.

The truth is that there is no such thing as a successful diet. That is the fact. The reality is that it is necessary to change our eating habits, for life. The only thing we can hang our hat on is change. In order for a person to survive in this 20th Century world, change must take place. Part of getting our act together emotionally, spiritually, and physically is to obtain a normal weight and keep it.

OVERWEIGHT AND OBESITY

Let me give you some statistics about people who are overweight and then we will discuss what we can do about it. If you are overweight, there is a 400% greater chance of diabetes and a 50% greater chance of heart disease. If you have a parent that is overweight, you have a 30% chance of being overweight. If you have two parents who are overweight, you have a 70% chance of being overweight. I feel that these odds of being overweight are due to the eating patterns of your parents that you saw and copied as a child rather than some genetic problem.

Jeffrey Bland, a noted biochemist, lists various problems due to obesity. He not only notes hypertension and increased risk of stroke, but impairment of cardiac function as well. He also names diabetes, liver disease, decreased glucose tolerance, insulin resistance, lung disease, problems with anesthesia during surgery, osteoarthritis, gout, endometrial cancer, abnormal lipid and lipoprotein metabolism as difficulties associated with obesity. Here are a few more statistics. Of children 18 and younger who are overweight, 80% will continue to be overweight as adults. Obesity begins to build up in childhood, when overeating increases the number of fat-containing cells. Studies of overweight children between 2 and 18 show that obese children have a greater number of fat cells than normal weight children of the same age, and unless diets are carefully controlled, the number of fat cells will continue to increase, never to disappear in adult years.

Diet pills are also not the answer. Not only do 90% of the people using diet pills regain their weight — 90%! — but there is also the danger of thinking that if one pill is good, two or more pills will be even better. Adverse reactions to the stimulants in these pills are serious, including high blood pressure, dizziness, even strokes and seizures — not to mention addiction.

- Thirty percent of 40-60 year olds are overweight. It is interesting that you do not see many elderly fat people. Either fat people lose weight in their later years, or they just don't live that long.

- Burning up the calories of a large apple requires 19 minutes of brisk walking. You need twice as much time for a candy bar.

- Obesity is rare in populations that consume fiber-rich high-carbohydrate diets.

- One hundred pounds of sugar is equivalent to 57 pounds of body fat — and remember that the average American eats 139 pounds of sugar per year. A diet rich in sugar and fat is more likely to lead to overconsumption of calories.

- Calorie counting does not take appetite and satiety into account. Eight ounces of refined sugar, like a candy bar, is equal to 2 1/2 pounds of beets or 20 average apples. Which would fill you up faster?

- No wild animal eats too much. It knows nothing of calories but does know appetite and the feeling of being full. There are no fat wild rabbits.

- Fluctuating weight also significantly increases the risk of premature death and heart disease. Findings suggest that you might be better off staying at a constant weight rather than watching the scales bounce up and down in continual lose/regain pattern. Researchers studied 5,127 people between 32 and 62 years of age. Their body weight was measured every two years. Results showed that people whose weight fluctuated frequently had twice the risk of dying of heart disease or other causes as those who kept their weight relatively stable. The health risks posed by repeated weight gain and loss may even exceed those of being overweight. The researchers suggest that if we are dieting and have lost weight, try to keep those pounds off.

- Those with upper body (stomach area) obesity are at greater risk of diabetes, hypertension and heart disease than those with lower-body (hip/buttocks area) obesity. I read a delightful poem in the Wall Street Journal one day recently which was an addendum to an article about this distinction. The poem was called "Shaping Up" by Marguerite Whitley May:

SHAPING UP

To add to the problems
With which we must grapple
It's better to look like
A pear than an apple
But if I could pick
A direction to lean,
I'd eschew the fruit
And become a string bean.

So What Can We Do?

Well, it probably will come as no surprise that I say it is balanced body chemistry that will help you lose weight and keep it off. Obesity means being out of balance — and if you can change your eating habits to bring about balance, your normal weight will find you. It won't happen quickly, and it won't happen without effort — you have to make a commitment to health and balance and you have to stick to it. This means eating reasonable to small portions of a variety of simple foods, keeping protein, fat, and sugar to a minimum.

Most dieters know that fat has twice as many calories per gram as carbohydrates and protein, but they usually concern themselves only with total calories. Dieters typically believe that they need a certain number of calories. If they consume more than that number, they gain weight. If they consume fewer, they lose. Simple, right? Wrong — as most dieters know only too well, it doesn't work.

I am not the only one who is saying that what you eat counts more than the calories: the American Heart Association, the American Cancer Society, and the Dietary Guidelines for Americans issued jointly by the Department of Agriculture and the Department of Health and Human Services, are saying the same thing. These organizations approach the issue from the disease prevention side: decrease your fat intake to reduce your risk of cancer and heart disease. The added benefit is that your weight should become much easier to control. The new message for dieters is "Don't focus on calories, and don't deprive yourself of complex carbohydrates — in fact, eat more carbohydrates."

If you are on Food Plan 3 for obesity or other health problems due to symptoms your body is giving you, you will know whether you are cheating because if you eat exactly like you are supposed to, you will lose weight. Remember, this includes monitoring your portion size — you can stay overweight on healthy foods if you eat enough of them! But if you are eating only the foods on Food Plan 3 in modest proportions and getting at least a little exercise every day, you will lose weight. If you do not lose weight you know you are cheating. It's that simple.

Remember, on this diet, which is really not a diet but an eating plan for the rest of your life, you can eat 5 or 6 times a day. Small amounts of food can be eaten often. But don't eat more than every two hours. I was 20 pounds overweight from the time I was 25 to 45 years old. Once I understood addictions, allergies, cravings and homeostasis, and got on this plan, I lost my weight and have kept it off.

Again, this is not a diet in the sense that you are going to lose weight and then go back to what you were eating. No. This is a plan for the rest of your life. For myself, I say that I am on Food Plan 3 all the time — and then I cheat now and then. How do I cheat?

Well, I don't eat sugar but I might eat too much food at one time, I might have some wheat which does not agree with me. I might have a barbecued chicken or I might have a glass of wine. And I do eat fruits between meals — although I didn't eat fruit while I was allowing my body to heal. While your body is healing you want to keep everything in homeostasis. Fruit, which is a simple sugar, will raise your blood sugar rapidly, and this is a stress for a body already worn down by illness. So remove all simple sugar, including fruit, for a few months to give your body its best chance to heal.

One of the reasons that I stay on Food Plan 3 is because I want to stay at 125 pounds, but more importantly, it is because I know I abused my body so much as a child and young adult by eating sugar, overeating, and eating fried foods, as well as being under a great deal of stress, and I was genetically born weak, therefore my body goes out of homeostasis easily and stays out longer than it should. Some people can cheat in their eating habits more than others and get away with it. Their body might become upset by something that they eat but they soon regain homeostasis. If you have ordered the body chemistry test kit (see page 168), you might try testing yourself after eating an abusive food, eating too much, or being under stress. See how long your body stays out of homeostasis. You might be surprised.

Exercise is important to all of us as part of a balanced program for health and wellbeing, but exercise is especially important in weight loss. Not only is it necessary for burning off calories, but exercise is also a great way to motivate yourself and keep your spirits high. And now there is some new research suggesting that exercising soon after eating is an efficient way to burn off excess calories.

The reason for this is that both eating a good meal and exercising raise your body's metabolic rate; therefore, you use up more calories exercising after a meal than before one. (Conversely, cutting back on calories lowers your metabolism and makes you work harder to burn off what you do eat.) The minimum requirement for working off a meal is a 20-minute walk within 45 minutes of eating. [From a study at the Division of Nutritional Sciences, Cornell University.]

There is a strong correlation between food cravings and obesity — which is no surprise to those of us who struggle with weight gain. We know that when we eat a certain food such as a bowl of ice cream, french fried potatoes, or even something as simple as a piece of cheese or an orange — we feel hungrier than before we ate the food. Some of us have urges for a particular food and find it hard to satisfy that craving unless we eat that particular food.

Whether you know it or not, you are allergy-addicted to that food. Just like a drug addict suffers withdrawal symptoms when the drug is withdrawn, allergic people experience discomfort when they do not eat a particular food. I'm sure a lot of you who are reading this can testify to the overwhelming power of food allergy-addiction. Compulsive eaters crave and continue to eat the foods to which they are addicted day after day. And we rarely have any idea that this daily food craving is based on a physiological need to stop the withdrawal symptoms that would occur if we did not repeatedly eat the food to which we are addicted. The phenomenon of simultaneous allergy and addiction to both foods and chemicals is discussed in Chapter 3. These allergy addictive foods, which are individual to each person, can cause chronic health problems such as obesity, migraine, fatigue, depression, and arthritis. An individual's genetic predisposition to allergies will then determine which part of his body will become the vulnerable target organ or tissue. Any major organ can become involved.

Water retention, or edema, is particularly common among allergic individuals and is an important contributing factor to obesity. Edema is the result of fluid retention due to an allergic response in the delicate, thin-walled capillary blood vessels present throughout the body. When the capillaries are temporarily injured during the course of an allergic reaction, body fluid passes through the capillary walls into the tissue surrounding the capillaries. The removal of an offending food will often result in a rapid water loss of 5 to 10 pounds within a week's time, all without the use of a diuretic.

Another problem with food allergies is that the allergic reaction itself can result in a drastic rise and then reduction in blood sugar with the accompanying symptoms of weakness, hunger, and irritability. The overweight person looks to eating to help his symptoms.

Normally our bodies have what we call an appestat. The appestat is that mechanism in the body which tells our brain when we have had enough food and we stop eating. Allergic hunger is pathological in that it does not respond to the normal satiety control center in the brain when food is consumed in normal amounts. So both the addictive and allergic responses to allergy can cause uncontrollable eating behavior.

Constipation is also a problem in many overweight people — as it is for many people who eat a standard American diet. Anyone who eats a lot junk food, food that has little fiber, such as white bread, sugar, white rice, and fried foods, instead of the complex carbohydrates that made up the majority of people's diets at the turn of the century, is likely to have a problem. So the same diet applies to people who are constipated as to people who are overweight — get on one of the healing food plans today. Do remember, you should have at least one bowel movement a day. If you do not have one bowel movement a day, think about adding fiber to your diet, and if necessary, occasionally try an herbal laxative.

Never take the laxatives that you find in regular drug stores. Remember that the small intestine is lined with villi, small finger-like projections of the intestinal lining that move in waves to push food along the digestive tract. Many commercial chemical laxatives irritate the villi, leading to their inflammation or even destruction. It is more difficult for us to digest our food when these villi have been irritated or shortened. So again, avoid chemical laxatives.

As you know I feel that soft drinks whether they have sugar in them or not, whether they have caffeine in them or not, should not be consumed. If you will read the fine print on the cans, you will see there is phosphoric acid in the drinks, whether or not they have sugar or caffeine. Consuming phosphoric acid changes the calcium phosphorus ratio and upsets all the minerals the same way sugar and other abusive foods do.

There is information that shows that diet soft drinks are not friends to dieters. This information is from an article is entitled "Sugarless Dieters." On any given day, one in four of us is on a diet. If you include artificial sweeteners and diet drinks in your battle of the bulge, your diet may be destined to fail. Doctors tracked 80,000 women in a six-year American Cancer Society study and found that women who were long-time users of artificial sweeteners put on excess pounds. Artificial sweetener users were far more likely to gain weight than women who didn't use sweeteners, and among women who gained weight, artificial sweetener users gained more than those who didn't use the products. It may be that women who use artificial sweeteners feel more justified in cheating on their diets. Another explanation may be that the artificial sweetener aspartame actually increases your appetite.

There is no good substitute for sugar. The best idea is to extract your sweet tooth. Remember, you are not on a diet but you are changing your eating habits and lifestyle both for balancing body chemistry and also losing weight.

Stress and Obesity

The relationship between stress and obesity is a logical one. I feel it is irrelevant which came first. I do know they go hand in hand. Some people can go on Food Plan 3, probably go through withdrawal symptoms for a few days, getting rid of their addictions. They not only eliminate lots of the allergies but also lots of stress. Other people can just deal with the psychological stress in their life and the foods and the inhalant allergies go away, and they also lose weight.

Research from Tufts University shows that young women who worry excessively about their weight are less likely to cope in a healthy way with negative experiences when they enter college. Shaky coping skills and unhealthy self-evaluation and eating patterns feed off each other making a cycle hard to break.

The body has to be treated holistically whether it be to balance body chemistry or to lose weight. Remember to check all four arenas, especially Arena I if you are having problems losing weight. You are responsible for what you put in your mouth. Many times your head gets in the way of your body losing weight: your body says "I don't need that candy bar" but your head says "Gimme, gimme!". It is up to you — you created a fat body and you can create a thin one. Just like you created an upset body chemistry, you can stop upsetting your body chemistry and let your mody find its natural healing mode.

Let me end this section with a few concrete suggestions you can apply as you change your eating habits for life — and lose that weight for life, too:

1. When you really really just want to EAT, go to the most expensive buffet you can find (the more expensive usually have the freshest food) and eat small portions from lots of different foods. This way you will pull from lots of different enzyme systems while eating a variety of foods.

2. Don't eat too much of one food because you will exhaust that enzyme system.

3. About an hour to one half hour before you eat a meal take the edge off of your hunger by drinking a tall glass of water. Sip it slowly, and it will give you a noncaloric first course that will help you to eat less at the meal.

4. Schedule your meals at fixed times every day, and stick to your routine as regularly as you can: breakfast at seven-thirty, lunch at twelve thirty and dinner at seven, as an example, or schedule four small meals a day. Your between-meal cravings will diminish as you reeducate your body to healthy eating patterns.

5. Consume as few calories as possible in liquid form because they go through the digestive tract faster than solid foods and will not be as satisfying. If you drink liquids other than water, try bouillon or tomato juice instead of fruit juices which have a lot of sugar.

6. Many clinics that treat people with weight problems have people use a cocktail fork rather than a dinner fork with which to eat.

7. Eat your salad first, and you can suppress your hunger while filling up on few calories.

8. Never allow yourself to become ravenous before you sit down to eat, or you'll definitely overeat. You'll eat more food and you'll eat it faster and taste it less. For that matter, avoid going food shopping hungry as well — that's how you end up with boxes of donuts in your pantry.

9. It is not necessary to scrape your plate clean. Always leave something on your plate, even just a scrap, as a tangible sign to yourself that you can quit when you choose.

10. If you find yourself wanting to eat more than you know you should, get up from the table, and go brush your teeth. Psychologically, having clean teeth will curb your desire to put more food in there, and physically, the toothpaste seems to soothe some of that sweet-craving. Also, be aware of the possible psychological basis of your cravings. When you have that sweet-craving, look to see what is not being fulfilled in your outer life that may be leading you to crave something to fill up the inside.

Natural healing takes time. You are not going on a diet for a few months, but you are going to change your pattern of eating — and thinking — for a lifetime.

OSTEOPOROSIS

Osteoporosis, the slow insidious loss of bone mass, is a weakening of the bone structure and a contributing factor in fractures, hip replacements, lower back pain, even death. Osteoporosis is a degenerative disease that begins slowly, for some in childhood, and for others in adulthood. In women, it often accelerates after menopause; in men, after age 65.

The people who are most prone to osteoporosis are post-menopausal women who are Caucasian and of Northern European descent. A composite high risk profile would be fair petite women who smoke and drink, take antacids, have a history in their family of osteoporosis, experienced menopause some years ago or had an early menopause, perhaps as a result of a hysterectomy. Thin people are more prone than obese — that is because fat cells have the ability to convert hormones secreted by the adrenal glands into estrogen. Also people who have taken corticosteroids or antibiotics over a long period of time are more prone to osteoporosis.

The main symptom of osteoporosis is loss of height, due to compression of the weakened vertebrae. Other symptoms are cramps in the legs and feet, bone pains, lower back pain, extreme fatigue, excess plaque on the teeth, and fractures of hips, spine, wrist or other parts of the skeleton. A patient rarely feels any pain until the fracture occurs. Dowager's hump (a forward bending of the upper spine), rickets, brittle or soft fingernails, and premature grey hair are also associated with osteoporosis — and therefore with calcium deficiency. However, it is usually not a matter of inadequate calcium intake but rather a problem of upset body chemistry that does not allow the available calcium to be properly utilized. There is more detail on this below.

Heart palpitations can be another sign of calcium deficiency. The medical community is treating some heart disease with calcium supplements and it is helping some, but it is not helping all people, because for some this calcium will become toxic, since it will not be usable by the body. And you can now understand why that is so, given that a balanced body chemistry is necessary in order to properly utilize any nutrients we take in.

What Causes Osteoporosis?

To explain this, I must first explain the composition of bones. Bones are basically made of three parts: 1) the compact outer layer called the cortical bone, 2) the spongy layer called the trabecular bone and 3) the marrow. Marrow is not destroyed, it is always with us. Cortical bone and trabecular bone are destroyed by cells called osteoclasts and made by cells called osteoblasts. When the cells are made it is called bone formation. When the cells are destroyed it is called bone resorption. When the body is getting all of its nutrients and is in balance, the osteoblasts will be working and our bones will be strong. When we are not metabolizing our nutrients or we are upsetting our body chemistry our osteoclasts will be overworking to keep a supply of calcium and other nutrients in the bloodstream and removing the calcium from the bones.

In your neck, lying at the front of the throat below the Adam's apple and just above the breastbone, is the thyroid gland. And at the base of the thyroid gland are four tiny glands called the parathyroid glands. These glands regulate the amount of calcium that is in your bloodstream. The bloodstream always wants to be in homeostasis or balance. If the level of calcium in the blood falls below a certain critical level, the parathyroid glands release parathyroid hormone into the bloodstream. The released hormone acts to increase the levels of calcium in your blood by doing three things. 1) It signals the kidneys to put calcium back into the blood stream. This is calcium that would have been excreted in the urine. 2) It stimulates the conversion of Vitamin D from an inactive to an active form, which allows the intestines to absorb more calcium from the foods you eat. 3) Most important of all, it stimulates the breakdown of bone, which in turn releases stored calcium into the blood stream. Calcium is so critical to life that your body is willing to sacrifice bone mass to ensure adequate levels in the blood stream.

As I said, the body always wants to be in homeostasis, in balance. This balancing act mediated by the parathyroid glands is a good example: when blood levels of calcium drop to a critical point, the mechanism pulls calcium from the bones, and when there is excess calcium in the bloodstream, the parathyroid gland helps to put the calcium back in the bones.

But, when you eat sugar, overcooked food, fried food, rancid fats, other abusive foods, or when you become distressed, you upset your body chemistry. The calcium increases in the blood stream — and the phosphorus decreases. A simple blood test will give this information, and you can order a kit for home use at the back of this book. Since minerals only work in relation to each other, when the phosphorus drops, the functioning calcium drops — even though there is extra calcium available (pulled from the bones because the body sensed an emergency situation); without its phosphorus partner, it can't be used by the body. This is why many sick people will show the optimal level of 9 to 10 1/2 mgs per deciliter of calcium in the blood stream even though their body is clearly behaving as though it were calcium deficient. The calcium might be there, but it cannot all function when other minerals in the body are deficient, because as I said, minerals only work in relation to each other.

Let's look at the other end now: When you eat sugar and the calcium level in your blood increases, where does that calcium come from? Chances are good that it is being pulled from your bones and tissues, since there is no calcium in sugar. The body is self-regulating; the mechanism wants to be balanced. So when there is extra calcium available, the mechanism is supposed to put calcium back into the bones. But when you eat abusive foods and distress yourself over and over, you are pulling more calcium out of your bones than you are putting back in and over a period of time, over decades, your bones lose their mass. This is osteoporosis.

It would seem logical just to take sufficient amounts of calcium to make sure you have enough, but unfortunately this will not always help. Let me explain why. Let's say a postmenopausal woman decides she needs 1200 milligrams of calcium per days so she drinks a milkshake which has 800 milligrams of calcium and a fruit yogurt which has 400 milligrams, for a total of 1200 milligrams of calcium. So everything is fine, right?

She is not only getting a heavy dose of calcium but also a heavy dose of sugar. A 12 oz. milkshake has 7 teaspoons of sugar and an 8 oz. cup of fruit yogurt has 7 teaspoons of sugar or honey in addition to the fruit. Therefore when you eat or drink these foods the sugar upsets your mineral relationships. Therefore, you could be consuming the correct amount of calcium but as long as you are upsetting your body chemistry, the calcium you are consuming may not be available for use, and can even become toxic to you. In fact, all that calcium in the shake and the yogurt can actually lead to pulling calcium from the bones rather than adding calcium to the bones.

Other 20th century life style factors pull calcium from the bones in the same way. Psychological stress, physical stress, excessive exercise, anorexia, too much protein, overcooking food, eating too much food at one sitting, caffeine, soft drinks (whether they contain sugar or caffeine or not), excess sodium, smoking, and alcohol all rob our bones of calcium.

Toxic minerals in our environment such as cadmium, lead, copper and zinc have been associated with bone loss in both farm animals and humans. Pharmaceutical drugs also leach calcium from our bones. The antibiotic tetracycline (which is also used to control acne), the blood thinner heparin, and corticosteroids all rob our bones of calcium. People who take antacids, such as Maalox and Mylantin, are more prone to osteoporosis, possibly because of the aluminum content in the antacids. Other over-the-counter drugs can also leach calcium from the bones.

From all the things we have talked about that can help to cause osteoporosis, you can see it is more important what you don't put in your mouth than what you do: don't put in sugar, too much protein, overcooked foods, antacids, alcohol, cigarettes, drugs products with aluminum or excess salt, because all these upset the body chemistry. When the body is in homeostasis, it has the opportunity to absorb more of the nutrients it needs from food. Incidentally, women who have severe rheumatoid arthritis are more likely to have osteoporosis than non-arthritic women of the same age. One of the factors is the long term use of corticosteroids, but even women with arthritis who have never used corticosteroid have lower bone mass.

Periodontal disease, also known as gum disorder or pyhorrea, is just osteoporosis of the mouth. If you lose bone in your mouth you can certainly lose bone in other parts of your body. Here are some interesting statistics about your teeth. 50% of the U.S. population over 65 have lost all their teeth. 25% of those over 55 have lost all their teeth. 60% of young adults (ages 20-34) have periodontal disease. 80% of middle-aged adults (35-54) have periodontal disease.

There is an interesting study correlating the relationship between periodontal disease and bone loss in the rest of the body. In a study of women between the ages 60 and 69, a definite correlation was observed between tooth loss and bone loss elsewhere in the body. Women with reduced cortical bone in fingers were more likely to have full or partial dentures than women with more cortical bone. Flossing the teeth, using the water pick, brushing three times a day and gargling with hydrogen peroxide are suggestions that dentists are giving people to prevent and/or stop periodontal disease. There is nothing wrong with these suggestions, but it is more important to stop upsetting your body chemistry. There are civilizations alive today that don't brush, floss, use a water pic, gargle or anything else and yet have no tooth decay or periodontal disease. They also eat their native foods and do not eat abusive ones.

How Can We Get Enough Calcium?

You might be surprised at how many foods contain significant amounts of calcium. Of course milk products have calcium in them, but many people get symptoms after they consume milk products. Again I must say that when the body is in homeostasis, it will absorb many more nutrients including calcium. There's lots of calcium in any fish that has bones, such as canned salmon, sardines or anchovies, and most other fish have a good amount of calcium as well. Dark green leafy vegetables such as spinach, collards, kale, parsley and turnip greens all are rich with calcium. Many other green vegetables, like broccoli and lettuce, have calcium also. The darker the lettuce the more the calcium — romaine has much more than iceberg. Soy beans have lots of calcium and can be eaten in the form of cooked soy beans, soybean milk, tofu or soy sauce. Do not expect to get much calcium from tofutti, the new dairyless ice cream, however. It does have the calcium but there's also honey or sugar. This upsets the body chemistry balance and makes all of the nutrients in tofutti less available to the body, including the calcium.

Almonds, pecans, Brazil nuts and all of the other nuts have calcium, and so do seeds — all seeds. A few other miscellaneous items that have heavy doses of calcium are oysters, kelp, and molasses (Barbados and Blackstrap). And last but certainly not least, a cup of carrot juice has as much calcium in it as a cup of milk and is much more digestible for many people.

Exercise is one of the most important factors in minimizing osteoporosis. As you have read, exercise is not just for toning your body and strengthening your heart. It also improves calcium absorption and stimulates bone formation. Exercise must be a regular part of your life. A daily 20 minute walk and some stretching and toning exercises 3 times a week is a minimum. In fact, exercise is the only way to significantly increase bone mass after you have stopped growing. As with muscles, stress on bones strengthens them. Activities that stress the long bones — walking, jogging, bicycling, rope jumping, tennis, basketball, and dancing send an electric current through the body that stimulates the growth, maintenance and repair of the skeleton.

Studies show that women who exercise for one hour 3 times a week for 1 year actually gained bone calcium while a comparison group of sedentary women lost calcium.Another study used 80 women volunteers between the ages of 35-65. These women played tennis 3 times a week. They were compared with 80 sedentary women. The tennis players in the 35 to 55 age group had little more bone than the control group, just as scientists had suspected because osteoporosis is uncommon before menopause, but the tennis players in the 55 to 65 age bracket had more bone than their control group. Without exercise, bedridden people tend to develop osteoporosis, as the bone minerals go in only one direction: into the blood plasma and out through the urine and stools rather than being reabsorbed in other bones. Exercise is something you should definitely not do without.

Arthritis and "Toxic" Calcium

When you upset your body chemistry and your phosphorus level drops, some of the calcium in your bloodstream becomes toxic because minerals only work in relation to each other. In this context, "toxic" means excess — and this excess, toxic calcium is part of the arthritic process. I spoke of this toxic calcium earlier. When your phosphorus level drops, you are simultaneously toxic in calcium (in other words, you have an excess of calcium, which will cause problems as I'll explain in a minute), and you also have a deficiency of functioning calcium. So your body does not read the information correctly. It continues to pull calcium from your bones and tissues, because it is looking for a balance of functioning calcium. And of course this continual pulling of calcium leads to osteoporosis. It is just that simple. Further, when you upset the minerals in the body, the mineral dependent enzymes cannot function as well. Therefore, all the food you eat does not digest properly. This undigested food gets into the blood stream. This is a form of food allergy and can cause havoc in the body. One of the places it can go is to the joints and tissues where it can cause arthritis. The joints and tissues become inflamed. The toxic calcium goes to these joints and tissues to try and help them. Unfortunately it doesn't do anything but make them stiff and sore.

Each arthritic is different. There are no particular foods that can be eliminated from the diets of arthritic people. The foods are individual to each person. For example, onions caused arthritis pain in the back of my neck. I was symptom free until I ate onions. When I did, it took from 12 to 24 hours for the pain to occur. At that time I could not move my neck easily from side to side or up and down. I was stiff and sore. If I did not eat any more onions I would be pain free in about two days. Onions do not upset every arthritic. It could be milk or wheat or anything else. Coffee is a common irritant for arthritics. The arthritic symptoms appear whether it be rheumatoid or osteoarthritis. I removed the onions completely for about two months, and I did not reintroduce them until I had no more pain. But during the two month healing phase, I had to watch very careful not to consume onions in any form in order to alleviate my allergy symptoms and in turn my arthritis.

If you are not taking any medications, you might try fasting for three days, either drinking only distilled water, or drinking just carrot and celery juice. The pain will subside, if you are not allergic to the carrots or celery. Hopefully you will become a believer in the principle that what you put in your mouth directly affects how you feel. During those three days you may have many symptoms, just like an alcoholic or drug addict has symptoms when he or she withdraws from alcohol or drugs. You might get headaches, perspiration, chills, fatigue, elevated temperature, or any other symptoms. When the toxic materials have left the body you will feel much better. When you end a fast or juice diet, take only steamed vegetables for your first meal. Add raw vegetables for your second meal. Do not eat protein until your third meal.

If you are taking medication, it is difficult to fast because you need to take your drugs with foods. In that case, I suggest you get on Food Plan 3 and start to identify the foods that upset your body chemistry.

HYPOTHYROIDISM

Although problems of the thyroid gland affect both men and women, they seem to be more of a problem for women. It is the thyroid gland, lying in front of the throat below the Adam's apple and just above the breastbone, which regulates the rate at which the body utilizes oxygen, and controls the rate at which various organs function, and the speed with which the body utilizes food.

The thyroid gland secretes a hormone into the blood stream called thyroxine. This hormone vies with insulin, a hormone secreted by the pancreas, to get into the cells. If your thyroid is not working correctly, there is a chance that your pancreas is also not working correctly. Just as minerals work in relation to each other, so do the endocrine glands work in relation to each other.

One way to check the functioning of the thyroid gland is to take your underarm temperature in the morning just before you get up. Shake the thermometer down the night before, then in the morning put it under one of your arms and keep it there for 10 minutes. Try this 2 or 3 mornings to make sure you are getting an accurate reading. If you are a menstruating woman, take your underarm temperature on the 2nd and 3rd day of your period. The reading should be 97.8 to 98.2. If it is lower or higher, you might read a book called Hypothyroidism, by Broda Barnes, M.D., or Solving the Riddle of Illness, by Stephen Langer, M.D., as well as checking with your doctor for a test for thyroid function. The best blood test for thyroid function tests the function of the thyroid stimulating hormone — the TSH test.

Here is another interesting bit of information concerning the thyroid. For some, even a slightly cool environment can lead to discomfort. They get cold quickly and warm up slowly. One reason may be that they are iron deficient. When two groups of women, one known to be anemic and the other non-anemic, were submerged up to their necks in water that was slightly cooler than body temperature, the iron-deficient women could not cope, and even the slight change of water temperature was unacceptable.

After 100 minutes, the anemic women had lower body core temperatures, produced less thyroid hormone and used less oxygen. This means that they were unable to accommodate the body's thermostat to external temperatures. Normal amounts of iron in the blood seem to increase thyroid output, raising the metabolic rate and increasing body temperature. So check your iron level. Raising the iron level might help with thyroid function.

The best way to help thyroid function is to put your body into homeostasis and let it heal. You will be amazed at what happens when you get on Food Plan 3. When the glands heal, they start secreting the right amount of hormone into the bloodstream and the hormone also gets into the cells and functions. This is true of all of the other glands too. Before I understood homeostasis, I was taking 7 grains of thyroid medication. Now that I am in balance most of the time, I take 2 grains. The body will heal as much as it is capable of. It just depends how much you have abused it, what you were genetically born with, how old you are, and how stressful your life is, as to how much it will heal. But you will be amazed.

⌇

HYPOGLYCEMIA AND DIABETES

As I have said, women tend to go to doctors more than men. Two of the diseases they get more than men are hypoglycemia and diabetes. From my experience women also eat more sugar than men, a great deal more sugar. If you haven't dealt with this problem and have some of the symptoms of unbalanced blood sugar, such as ravenous hunger three or four hours after you eat sugar, perspiration, dizziness, lightheadedness, fatigue and/or shakiness after meals, I suggest that you immediately get on Food Plan 3 for two months to give your pancreas a chance to heal. Remember that Food Plan 3 does not include fruits. If you are sugar sensitive, you could be sensitive to fruit also, because there is enough simple sugar in fruit to upset your body chemistry like sugar does. Although fruit is not what causes the problem, it can continue the problem. Use the body chemistry test kit to check for food allergies, since they can raise and lower the blood sugar just like sugar. For instance, eggs used to make my blood sugar too high. This is interesting, since eggs contain no simple sugar and yet they made my blood sugar go up. I think my pancreas was confused.

The Glucose Tolerance Test

I do not recommend that anyone take the glucose tolerance test. I feel that taking 100 milligrams of sugar on an empty stomach is a giant invasion to your body. I have counseled people who were never the same after they had the glucose tolerance test. Usually the people who take the test are not well to begin with, they have upset body chemistry to begin with. Their homeostatic mechanisms are not working well to begin with. Then they take this sugar water and their homeostatic mechanisms have to adapt to 100 milligrams of sugar being poured into their body. Do check with your doctor for some alternatives to this test. There are alternative methods to test for hypoglycemia and diabetes. Check with different doctors for these methods.

If you do have the test and they diagnose either high or low blood sugar, chances are you will be put on a diet very similar to my Food Plan 3. If your doctor doesn't put you on such a diet, ask some questions! I suggest that you forget the test and just get on the diet if you have the symptoms.

Hypoglycemia, or low blood sugar, is an easy problem for most people to solve. When the body is put back in balance, the pancreas will start secreting the right amount of insulin and the symptoms will go away, if you are not upsetting your body in any other way.

Diabetes is more complicated. There are basically two types of diabetes. Type 1 is childhood onset diabetes. In this form, the pancreas is unable to secrete any insulin. This is a more difficult type of diabetes to manage than Type 2, and almost always requires medication.

Type 2 diabetes, called adult onset diabetes, is different from Type 1 because insulin is secreted from the pancreas but it is unable to function properly. For many people, once the body is put back into homeostasis, the insulin will have a much better chance to function.

I have seen people with both Type 1 and Type 2 diabetes lower their insulin requirements tremendously when their body chemistry has been regained and maintained. There is a book called Victory over Diabetes, written by Dr. William Philpott, which I recommend that every hypoglycemic and diabetic read.

It is important for diabetics and hypoglycemics to remove simple sugars from their diets for at least a period of two months to give the pancreas a chance to heal and function properly. As I have said, enzymes are dependent upon minerals to function. Each enzyme depends on a certain mineral or minerals in order to do its work. Phosphoglutamase is an enzyme used to digest simple sugars. It is chromium dependent. Research shows that hypoglycemics and diabetics are deficient in chromium. Taking extra chromium is not the answer. The answer lies in not upsetting your body chemistry and letting the chromium you do get from your foods function properly.

CANDIDA ALBICANS

Candida is an organism that lives in all of our bodies but seems to overgrow in more and more women and men today. It is a normal flora in our bodies, a simple form of yeast. When we have a balanced body chemistry and a strong immune system it lives happily within us, but when we upset our minerals and have a low concentration of functioning calcium, our immune system cannot keep *Candida* in balance and it overgrows.

As we said earlier, part of our immune system consists of the phagocytes that gobble up foreign invaders. In a fasting state, each phagocyte is able to deal with 16 foreign invaders like bacteria, viruses, and undigested food. But when we drink a Coke or eat sugar in some other form, the phagocytes become inefficient — they can only handle 3 or 4 foreign invaders each. This is one way the *Candida* can overgrow.

I might also add that at the time you drink the Coke, if there is bacteria in your mouth or throat, because your phagocytes are inefficient, you are more likely to get the disease. It takes between 2 and 4 hours for the phagocytic index to come back to normal after drinking Coke; during that time you are far more susceptible to disease. The average person drinks 560 soft drinks a year; of those 380 contain sugar. A lot of people drink 3 or 4 soft drinks a day and keep their immune system depressed all the time.

As I said, *Candida* is an organism. It has to eat and excrete, just like we do, but it doesn't have a toilet, so it defecates inside of us. There are 72 different things in the *Candida* feces that we can react to. If we compromise our immune system we will not have the ability to handle the 72 different items in the feces, so all that our immune system does is react to the 72 different things. We think we are victims of the *Candida* but we have forced it to overgrow by feeding it. *Candida* loves sugar but it also likes wine and all alcohol. If you have symptoms of food allergies as well as bloating, fatigue, vaginal discharge or dry eyes, you might remove all simple sugars from your diet — *Candida* loves them.

That includes fruit which has lots of simple sugars. Also watch out for fermented foods like vinegar, soy sauce, and tofu. I recommend that you read *The Yeast Connection* by Dr. William Crook and *Candida: A Twentieth Century Disease* by Dr. Shirley Lorenzani. Also avoid the birth control pill, corticosteroids and antibiotics. *Candida* seems to thrive on all of these. *Candida* also proliferates in a person who is in distress, a person who is angry, depressed, in rage or who holds judgments against other people.

With *Candida*, one stress on the body leads to another and in turn leads to another. If you have excess *Candida*, you must address all areas of your life in order to get well. You may need to detoxify your body by going on a carrot and celery juice diet for three or four days. Then go on Food Plan 3. This diet consists of combining small amounts of five or six vegetables with small amounts of protein from fish, chicken, eggs or red meat or from combining beans and grains.

The good news is that *Candida* has a difficult time proliferating in a healthy body. Address all four arenas as discussed in Chapter 5, avoid sugar and abusive foods, and keep your body in balance, and *Candida* will not be a problem for you.

⌒

THE UNIVERSAL REACTOR: SEVERE ENVIRONMENTAL SENSITIVITY

Your immune system can be challenged by a variety of things, and when there are too many challenges at once, your immune system can become both overloaded and hyperactive. If your immune system is put under that kind of stress long enough, you may become what I call a "universal reactor" — developing allergies to just about everything in your environment: chemicals, foods, dust, mold, and pollen, for instance. If this is your situation, you need to take drastic action:

1. Get on Food Plan 3.

2. Use the Body Chemistry Kit to identify the particular foods that you react to.

3. Wash all your food carefully.

4. Go on an anti-*Candida* regime, taking acidopholus and caprillic acid. Read the *Candida* section above.

5. Use the Four Arena guidelines. Each of us is a unique individual and each responds differently to a variety of therapies. For some people simple modifications in lifestyle can greatly improve health. Other people need to explore many different modalities in order to give the body a chance to heal.

☞

THE SPECIAL HEALTH NEEDS OF WOMEN

In this section, I will talk about three specific conditions that affect "women only" — PMS, menopause, and the Pill.

PMS

Let me start by telling you what PMS is and giving you some interesting facts about it. PMS is a collection of symptoms - any combination of emotional or physical features that occur cyclically. 45% of pre-menopausal women have some symptoms. 120 million working days are lost annually in Great Britain due to this problem. When violent crimes were committed by women, 62% were in the pre-menstrual week compared to 2% in the week after. Shoplifting is 30 times more common in the second half of the menstrual cycle than in the first half. 53% of women's suicide attempts occur during day 20 to 28 in a woman's cycle. These statistics are certainly indicative that women feel better at certain times of the month than others.

PMS symptoms can be divided into four categories: pain, edema, emotional symptoms, and other. Examples of pain are — cramps, headaches, backaches, muscle spasms and breast tenderness. Symptoms of edema or swelling include weight gain, pelvic pressure, joint swelling, bloating and breast swelling. Emotional symptoms include anxiety, tenseness, argumentativeness, and fear of losing control. Other symptoms include nausea, acne, insomnia and dizziness.

I am not a doctor and I do not diagnose, but I have seen women in pain with PMS. And often, when their fallopian tubes were blown with air to clear any clogging, their pain also went away. If you have pain in your lower abdomen premenstrually, I certainly would check with a doctor to see if that is a problem. I had severe cramps almost from the onset of my period at age 14 until I tried to get pregnant. I would become nauseated, throw up, perspire and generally feel miserable for about four hours and then it would pass. After the doctors blew my tubes clean when I was trying to get pregnant, the pain stopped, and has not returned. I certainly wish I had known the body chemistry principle at that time because I would have saved myself lots of pain by not upsetting my body chemistry so often and so long as I had been doing. Abdominal pain is only one symptom of PMS.

Food cravings also play a role with women who have PMS. It has been found that low blood sugar (hypoglycemia) is often a major contributing factor. One simple control method for PMS patients with hypoglycemia is eating between six to eight small meals a day to help maintain appropriate blood sugar levels. Eat small meals from Food Plan 3. New research shows that nibbling all day rather than eating the traditional "three squares" also lowers cholesterol and blood pressure.

Overweight can also be a problem. Virtually all women who suffer from PMS are prone to edema, or fluid retention. Diuretics, also called water pills, do not always work and they can create new problems such as longterm critical deficiencies in potassium and magnesium. Edema is not always simple retention; sometimes it is actually a fluid shift from one area of the body to other areas, such as to the abdomen, and there is no real weight gain. Some vitamin pills such as vitamin B6, up to 500 milligrams a day, and vitamin C, 1 gram or more twice a day, act as diuretics. Distilled water in itself will act as a diuretic if taken in sufficient quantities. Those who do persist in taking diuretics other than from a natural source certainly should eat foods high in potassium such as bananas, dates, eggs, peaches, tomato juice, seafood, nuts, potatoes and chicken. Another valuable supplement is magnesium. Study tests show that, in severe PMS, the red blood cells are deficient in magnesium which may help to account for the salt craving experienced by many women. Good food sources of magnesium are whole grains, green leafy vegetables, legumes, nuts, cereals and shellfish. Calcium metabolism is also involved in this highly interactive nutrition team. The newest research shows that some PMS can be alleviated by taking two times as much magnesium as calcium a week before your menstruation begins until the day it begins. During the other time in your cycle just take equal amounts of calcium and magnesium.

Another frequently used supplement for PMS patients is kelp. The second half of the menstrual cycle is strongly affected by thyroid function. If you show a low underarm temperature in the morning when you wake up, I suggest that you first try some extra iodine and/or kelp as well as balancing your body chemistry for a month before you see a doctor for prescription thyroid medication.

And remember that all of these remedies are only necessary while your body is healing. After two months of a balanced body chemistry, the symptoms should go away.

PMS is an imbalance in the body chemistry, specifically of the endocrine system. The glands of the endocrine system secrete hormones into the blood stream. The pancreas secretes insulin, the adrenals secrete adrenaline, the thyroid secretes thyroxin among others. When we suppress our minerals, our glands are not going to work as well. Some glands might secrete more than their share of hormone as Melvin Page explained in his book, *Your Body is Your Best Doctor*. If you are genetically programmed with an endocrine system that does not function optimally and then abuse it through lifestyle, during the time of hormonal changes in the body, the body is more likely to have problems. Your body will start giving signals that all is not well.

Many of these symptoms can be caused by other health problems also but when they occur cyclically then chances are they are related to the menstrual cycle.

In my practice I have seen all of these symptoms disappear in as little as two menstrual cycles when a woman gets on the program and stops upsetting her body chemistry. It truly is that easy. I wish I had had this information when I was young because some months I would throw up for three or four hours at a time. I also was consuming an incredible amount of sugar and abusing my body in other ways as well.

As I have said, some of us are born genetically stronger than others. The strong people can abuse their bodies more and get away with it and not have symptoms. If you were genetically born weak and you abuse your body, you will be more susceptible to symptoms as well as degenerative diseases. So the PMS of today can become another health problem in the future.

Menopause

Menopause can be a time of physical disturbance and mental disturbance in a woman's life. It is not only a time of hormonal change, but often is a time of great physical and emotional change as well. Perhaps your children are leaving home and your day to day emotional involvement with them is suddenly gone. If you are not working outside the home, your work load may suddenly be very different — and all that time on your hands may not seem like a blessing. Eating patterns in your household can change when there is no longer a large family to cook for. So not only is your body going through a change but also your day to day routine is changing. As Alvin Tofler said in his book, Future Shock, when we go through too many changes at one time we become more susceptible to diseases. In body chemistry terms, too much change can turn normal stress into distress, and distress causes upset body chemistry. Upset body chemistry suppresses the immune system, takes you out of the natural healing mode, and invites disease.

Life is a process of coping, life is not letting stress become distress. There are some things you can do to lower the stress load and help the body to take its natural course through menopause.

The first thing to do is to take care of yourself. Make sure that you take time for yourself. Make sure that you maintain or regain your normal weight. Make sure to continue to have a good sex life. Take time in your life to have fun. If you do not have a sport that you love, try a new one. Take instructions in golf, tennis, archery or something else of your choice. Exercise is very important at this time in life. Hopefully you have been exercising forever, but if you have not, now is the time to start.

Make sure your clothes fit and look well on you. Is your environment a good place to live and/or work in? If it is not, make it into an environment that you are comfortable in — clean the carpets, buy a new throw rug, put up new drapes, paint your walls, or straighten up your shelves. Do you have a support system? Do you have friends you can call? If you don't, there are many groups to join: tennis clubs garden clubs, health clubs, singles groups, local theater or singing groups, hiking clubs, square dancing — just about any activity is likely to have a group that developed around it. Check your local newspapers. I truly think that mental and physical health requires a holistic approach. Get your whole act together. Life is too short to waste it on things you do not like to do. If you find yourself in this position, try to eliminate some of those things you do not like to do. Make the second half of your life better than the first.

Research from the University of Alabama shows that menopause is less distressing and presents fewer emotional and physical problems and symptoms for women who have a clear purpose in life. Three personality traits to help obtain a purpose are assertiveness, independence and authoritativeness.

Estrogen replacement therapy is another controversial topic. What I will say is that there may be good reasons to take estrogen for some women, particularly those who go through menopause early, whether due to hysterectomy or other reasons. am not a medical doctor and I feel that this is a topic best left to the medical profession, but I will say that the more you upset your body chemistry, the more susceptible you will be to menopause symptoms. For instance, you will be more likely to secrete calcium in your urine and therefore be more prone to osteoporosis. Whether you take estrogen or not, it is important to balance your body chemistry.

I will say that I have just recently been through menopause and found that as long as I kept myself in homeostasis, I had a minimum of symptoms. When your body is in balance and then goes through hormonal changes, it is much easier on your body. I found that taking extra Vitamin E helped me. As you know, I do not believe in magic pills and a lot of pills do not make a magic potion. Since I was not upsetting my body chemistry, I took 1200 International Units of Vitamin E. If you are not taking Vitamin E now, start with 400 a day for a week, then 800 a day for a week and then 1200. Also remember to take a multiple vitamin and mineral during this time, in fact all the time. Once the symptoms go away, drop the Vitamin E to 400 I.U.s.

Our body processes will get slower as we age, but I do not believe that that has to mean less quality in your life. If you do not wake up happy and go to bed happy most every day, find out why — and change it. There are so many ways to get psychological help. Each one of us must find our own path. I spent many years doing psychoanalysis, Scientology, working with Elizabeth Kubler-Ross, doing Jungian therapy, writing in a journal and having body work done. Your path will be your own. But don't quit until you do wake up happy and go to bed happy. Health is a right, not a privilege. Fight for that right.

The Birth Control Pill

I recently read an article in the *Los Angeles Times* about research that showed the birth control pill did not have any direct effect on uterine cancer, breast cancer or heart disease. I am sure that this research is valid. I'm glad to hear that good news, but what the research didn't say is what the pill does to adversely affect the health of many women. The article concerned itself only with the positive aspects of the pill, but as far as I'm concerned there are enough negative aspects to think twice — or three times — before you take the pill.

Here is a list of women who are at high risk for medical problems if they take the pill:

- Women who have a history of blood clots or slow-moving blood

- Women who smoke

- Women who have frequent headaches

- Women who tend to retain fluid.

And frankly, I'm not sure that the average woman who has no symptoms should be taking it either. I have seen enough women in my practice who have been on the pill in the past and/or who are on it now who have a problem with yeast, *Candida albicans*. These people suffer the normal symptoms of *Candida* over-growth: bloating, fatigue and food allergies. They might or might not have the vaginal discharge and itching. All of the symptoms of *Candida* are eliminated or alleviated when they no longer take the pill. *Candida* is a big problem for women on the pill, particu-larly if they continue to eat sugar, have taken antibiotics or corti-costeroids, or are under a great deal of stress, because all of this can cause an overgrowth of yeast.

Another problem with the pill is that it interferes with the absorption of vitamins B12, B6, C and folic acid. It can also dis-turb the critical hormonal balance of the body. I have seen many women with enlarged breasts while on the pill, and within a period of 6 weeks after they stop taken the pill, their breasts go back to normal size. These symptoms in themselves are scary, but what is actually going on in the body needs to be addressed too. Each woman has to decide for herself what is the best con-traceptive to use. I certainly think that this needs to be discussed with your partner and your doctor. Find all the information you can in both the traditional medical field and the holistic field before you decide to take the pill on a long term basis.

☞

THE GOOD NEWS

Each one of us can stop the degenerative disease process and let the body heal. Your body symptoms can go away and you can die of old age, not in pain with arthritis or osteoporosis, not of heart disease or cancer — just old age.

Our 20th Century lifestyle is a problem for many of us. If you have no symptoms, no fatigue, take no drugs, have no lower back pain, have lots of energy, then then your body still has the ability to regain homeostasis quickly. You are lucky, but I agree with Dr. Hans Selye who believes that we have only a limited amount of reserves. When we abuse our body long enough, we use up the reserves until eventually we no longer have the ability to regain and maintain homeostasis. My best advice to you is to try to continually keep your body in balance, in its natural healing mode. That is when it will function best for you — now and in the future.

All the diseases of which I have spoken have one thing in common. We have done something to our body to cause these diseases. Some of us are unfortunate enough to have more than one of these problems. But in all cases, the answer is: Stop doing to your body what you did to make it sick — and the body will heal itself.

CHAPTER 7

Recipes

The following recipes are just a tiny sampling of the many delicious dishes you can enjoy while on Food Plan 3 for maximum healing. The first section contains main dish recipes gathered from friends, favorite restaurants, and my earlier books. The next section, sweetness without sugar, is for those of you who can't imagine a life without sugar. It contains selections from my own recipes using only the foods from Food Plan Three.

Experiment with these recipes and then create your own. Be adventuresome! Good, fresh, wholesome food doesn't need to be complicated or expensive. Learn about the fruits and vegetables that are native to your region and substitute as needed. A lifetime of healthful eating awaits you!

Main Dishes

⌒

Ginger Chicken Salad

This recipe is unusual because of the contrast of the warm chicken with the cool salad vegetables.

> 1/4 cup Ginger Dressing (see next page)
>
> 2 tablespoons sesame seeds, optional
>
> 2 tablespoons butter
>
> 1 clove garlic, minced
>
> 1 inch cube ginger, grated
>
> 3 half chicken breasts, deboned
>
> 2 tablespoons water
>
> 3 cups lettuce, torn
>
> 1 cup Chinese cabbage, slivered
>
> 1 cup parsley, chopped
>
> 1 cup celery, sliced
>
> 1/4 cup green onions, sliced
>
> 1/2 cup red cabbage, slivered

Prepare Ginger Dressing (see below) and let sit. Spread sesame seeds out on a pan and toast in a 250° F. oven about 30 minutes. Melt butter over low heat and sauté garlic and ginger. Cut chicken into bite-sized pieces and sauté in butter. Add water, cover pot and cook chicken over low heat until done. Chop vegetables into salad bowl. Add hot chicken to salad. Pour Ginger Dressing over salad and toss. Sprinkle hot sesame seeds over salad and serve at once. Makes 4 servings.

Variations:

Cooked peas, avocado cubes, or 1 cup cooked rice may be added.

Cooked turkey can be sautéd for a few minutes and substituted for chicken. Try fish for contrast.

Red onion rings can be substituted for red cabbage.

Ginger Dressing

3 tablespoons olive oil

1 to 2 tablespoons lemon juice

1 teaspoon freshly grated ginger

1 clove garlic

Mix and let sit a few minutes. Pour over salad or cooked vegetables. Makes 1/4 cup.

From *The Candida Albicans Yeast-Free Cookbook*. The Price Pottenger Nutrition Foundation, 2667 Camino del Rio So. #109, San Diego, CA 92108.

Lentil Tomato Loaf

2 cups cooked lentils

2 cups canned tomato sauce

1/2 cup chopped onion

1/2 cup chopped celery

3/4 cups oats

1/2 teaspoon garlic powder

1/4 teaspoon Italian seasoning

1/4 teaspoon celery seeds

1/2 teaspoon salt

1/4 teaspoon pepper

Combine all ingredients in a large bowl. Pack into an oiled 9x5 inch loaf pan. Bake at 350° F. for 45 minutes. Let cool slightly before unmolding. Makes 4 servings.

From *Lick the Sugar Habit,* Nancy Appleton. Garden City Park, New York: Avery Publishing Co., 1988. Used by permission.

Molded Chicken Salad

3 cups cooked rice

2 cups cooked chicken, chopped

1 cup cooked green peas

1 cup celery, chopped

1/2 cup green onions (including tops), thinly sliced

1/4 cup pimentos, chopped

2 envelopes unflavored gelatin

1/2 cup double-strength chicken broth (cold)

2/3 cup mayonnaise

1 tablespoon lemon juice

2 teaspoons salt

1 teaspoon seasoned pepper

In a large mixing bowl combine rice, chicken, peas, celery, onions, and pimentos. Soften gelatin in broth; heat to dissolve, and combine with mayonnaise, lemon juice, salt, and pepper. Add to rice mixture and mix thoroughly.

Spoon into a 1-1/2 quart mold or individual molds. Chill until set. Unmold onto salad greens, if desired. Makes 6-8 servings.

From *Healthy Bones*, Nancy Appleton. Garden City Park, New York: Avery Publishing Co., 1991. Used by permission.

Crunchy Chopped Salad with Shrimp

1 pound Florida rock shrimp

1 clove garlic, minced

2 teaspoons olive oil

2 cups fresh corn, cut off the cob

2 Hass avocados, diced

1 cup jicama, diced

1/4 cup diced radish

1/4 cup diced red pepper

1/4 cup diced green onion

1/4 cup chopped cilantro

1 head romaine lettuce, shredded

Pat the shrimp dry. Heat the garlic in the olive oil in a 12" skillet over medium heat until fragrant. Add the shrimp and sauté until cooked through, approximately 4 minutes. Set aside to cool.

Toss the cooled shrimp with the lime cumin dressing (below) and all the remaining ingredients except the lettuce. Arrange the lettuce on a serving platter and top with the shrimp mixture. Makes 4 servings.

Courtesy of Teri Appleton Villanueva, Chef and Cooking Teacher, Los Angeles, California.

Lime Cumin Vinaigrette

1/4 cup olive oil

3 tablespoons freshly squeezed lime juice

1 teaspoon ground cumin

1 small jalapeno, seeded and minced

1/2 teaspoon salt

1/4 teaspoon black pepper

Whisk all ingredients together in a small bowl.

Lentil and Vegetable Stew

1/4 cup olive oil

1 cup onion, coarsely chopped

1/2 cup celery, coarsely chopped

1/2 cup carrot, coarsely chopped

2 tablespoons minced garlic

2 cans (35 oz. each) whole peeled tomatoes, pureed

6 cups chicken stock or water

1/2 cup lentils

1/2 cup zucchini, coarsely chopped

1/2 cup yellow squash, coarsely chopped

1/2 cup peas, fresh or frozen

1/2 cup corn, fresh or frozen

1/2 teaspoon crushed red pepper flakes

2 teaspoons salt

1 teaspoon black pepper

1 cup chopped parsley

In a large stockpot, heat the olive oil. Sauté the onion and celery until translucent. Add the garlic and carrots and sauté until fragrant. Add the pureed tomatoes, chicken stock, and lentils. Bring to a boil, then reduce heat and simmer for 20 minutes. Add the remaining ingredients and simmer approximately 30 minutes more. Serves 4 to 6.

Quinoa-Vegetable Salad

2 cups quinoa, roasted then washed

3 cups water

1/4 teaspoon sea salt

4 ribs of celery, diced

2 ears corn, shaved off the cob

2 red bell peppers, diced

2 medium carrots, diced

1 medium zucchini, diced

4 scallions, thinly sliced on the diagonal

3 tablespoons fresh dill

Wash the quinoa carefully, then dry roast in a cast-iron skillet until you smell a nutty aroma and see the quinoa has become brown and toasty.

Bring water to a boil in a small wide-mouth pot, pour in the quinoa and turn the heat down to a simmer. In about 20 to 25 minutes, the quinoa will be done. Take a fork and fluff it while removing it from the pot into a bowl. Let it cool.

Lightly blanch the vegetables, drain, and let cool.

Toss grain with veggies and fresh dill and chill.

Serve on a bed of red leaf and romaine with a touch of red cabbage, carrots, and alfalfa sprouts. Makes 4 servings.

Courtesy of Ann Gentry, Proprietress, Real Food Daily, 514 Santa Monica, Santa Monica, California.

Mexican Corn Soup

Chunks of sweet corn give this savory soup richness and texture. For a zestier flavor, add more red pepper sauce.

Prep Time: 20 minutes • Cooking Time: 30 minutes

> 1 teaspoon olive oil
>
> 1 cup onion, finely chopped
>
> 2 tablespoons whole cumin seeds
>
> 8 cups corn, fresh or frozen
>
> 5 cups vegetable stock
>
> 1 tablespoon salt
>
> pinch black pepper
>
> 6 tablespoons tomato paste
>
> 1 cup soy milk
>
> 1/2 teaspoon red pepper sauce
>
> 1/2 bunch fresh cilantro, minced

In large soup pot, heat oil. Add onion and cumin seeds and cook for five minutes until onions are translucent. Add corn, stock, salt, pepper, and tomato paste. Puree half the soup in a blender, then return soup to the pot and stir well to combine. Add soy milk and red pepper sauce and reheat without boiling. Simmer 25 minutes. Makes 6 to 8 servings. Adjust seasonings to taste and add fresh cilantro, if desired.

Courtesy of Grassroots Natural Market and Kitchen, 1119 Fair Oaks Avenue, South Pasadena, CA.

Becky's Fajitas

1-1/2 pounds chicken, sliced into strips and marinated for 2 hours (recipe below.) (Slightly freezing chicken will make it easier to slice.)

3/4 tablespoon oil

1/2 cup sliced onion

1/2 cup green onion, chopped (or 1 cup zucchini strips)

1 cup sliced red bell pepper

2 avocados, peeled and sliced

Salsa

Lettuce

Cooked brown rice

Quickly sauté onions (or zucchini) and peppers in oil until lightly browned. Remove from pan. Sauté marinated chicken about 4 minutes, then toss with vegetables. Make into a salad with the lettuce, avocados, and the amount of rice you desire. Makes 6 servings.

Marinade:

1 clove garlic, minced

1-1/2 teaspoons seasoned salt (sugar and yeast free)

1/4 teaspoon chili powder

1/4 teaspoon crushed red pepper

2 tablespoons oil

2 tablespoons lemon juice

Combine all ingredients and mix well.

From *Get Healthy Cookbook*, Bessie Jo Tillman, M.D. Redding, CA: Enjoy, 1991. (Box 4726, Redding, CA 96099.)

Provincial Ratatouille

1 eggplant, peeled and thinly sliced

1 zucchini, sliced likewise

1 small onion, chopped

2 garlic cloves, finely minced

1/2 can tomato paste

1/2 can chicken broth

4 tablespoons olive oil

2 sprigs fresh basil, chopped

2 sprigs fresh parsley, chopped

Sprinkle the eggplant and zucchini with olive oil and sauté in a very hot pan until slightly tender. Set aside, allow to cool, then cut into smaller bits. Makes 4 servings.

Sauté the onion to translucency, then add the garlic. After a minute, add the tomato paste, chicken broth, eggplant and zucchini. Simmer for a few minutes then sprinkle with basil and parsley. Delicious hot or chilled.

Dilly Carrot Soup

2 cups chicken broth

2 cups water

2 pounds carrots, chopped

1 cup fresh raw carrot juice

1 onion, chopped

1 celery stalk, chopped

2 cloves garlic, minced

2 cups garden peas (fresh or frozen)

2 large sprigs fresh dill, chopped

- or -

2 tablespoons dried dill

In your favorite soup pot, mix broth and water and bring to boil. Reduce heat and add carrots, onion, celery, and garlic. When all is tender, remove a cup of the carrots and set aside. Puree remainder in blender or processor, then pour back into the pot, adding the peas, dill, the set-aside carrots, and raw carrot juice.

At the last minute, fearlessly stir in 2 tablespoons of fresh raw cream. (For most people, cream is okay while milk, yogurt, cream cheese, and sour cream may aggravate allergies.)

Sweetness Without Sugar

I have made these recipes for people who are allergic to wheat and milk products, and want to eat sugar free. If you can tolerate butter, chances are you can tolerate small amounts of whipping cream, which is mostly butter. I rarely indicate more than one tablespoon of whipping cream per serving.

As for desserts, many people who are allergic to foods are sugar-sensitive. Many have yeast infections (*Candida albicans*), hypo-glycemia, or are pre-diabetic. While a body is healing itself of its allergies, all simple sugars should be avoided, even fruit. This means life without sugary desserts, which for sugarholics can be catastrophic. Our challenge is to create wheat-free, milk-free dishes with no sugar, no chemical sugar substitutes, no fruits, and no fruit juices.

As I believe these recipes will show you, the challenge is easily met. I hope you will be inspired to experiment and create your own.

Coconut Yam Souffle

1 large yam (about 2 cups), steamed

1/2 cup coconut milk

1 teaspoon grated lemon rind

1/2 cup shredded coconut, toasted

2 eggs

1 teaspoon vanilla extract

While steaming the yam (or sweet potato), separate the yolks from the whites and beat the whites until stiff. When the yam is tender, let it cool slightly before peeling and mashing with coconut milk, lemon rind, and egg yolks until fluffy. Add the vanilla. Salt to taste. Then, fold the egg whites thoroughly into the mixture, and pour into a 7" soufflé dish. Bake in preheated 350° oven for 40 minutes.

This delightful invention enhances all forms of meat dishes as a side dish, but it is best as a sugarless dessert, especially if you spoon on an interesting sauce made of three parts coconut milk well stirred with one part blackstrap molasses. Makes 4 servings.

Non-Allergic Holiday Pie

For one pastry shell, sift:

> 1/2 cup barley flour
>
> 1/2 cup quinoa flour
>
> 1/2 cup millet flour (any other flour such as rice, bean, etc. will work also, just use 1/3 of each)
>
> 1 teaspoon aluminum free baking powder

Cut in: 6 tablespoons butter

Add: 1/4 cup ice water (approximate)

Mix together gently by hand until it forms a ball. Roll out on floured cutting board, place in pie pan, trimming edges. Bake at 400° for 10-12 minutes.

Filling:

> 3 large sweet potatoes
>
> 1 teaspoon vanilla
>
> 1/2 teaspoon cinnamon
>
> 1/2 teaspoon nutmeg
>
> 1/2 teaspoon allspice
>
> 1/2 cup heavy cream

Bake or steam the sweet potatoes until very tender. Peel, then mash with cream until fluffy, blending in the spices. Place in pie crust and serve warm or cold. Can also be served as a parfait in champagne glasses, with a modest topping of whipped cream. Makes 6 servings.

Carob Mousse

3 large sweet potatoes

1/2 cup carob power (or to taste)

1 teaspoon vanilla (or to taste)

1/2 cup heavy whipped cream

Bake or steam the sweet potatoes until tender. Peel and fluff with carob powder and vanilla. Blend well. Whip cream and fold gently into mixture, blending well. Spoon into champagne glasses or demitasses. Chill and serve cold. Makes 6 servings.

Scones

Scones are an English version of the American biscuit. They are a little lighter. Having spent time in England, I fell in love with scones and learned how to make them without sugar or wheat. But be careful, they are addictive!

1/3 cup barley flour

1/3 cup millet flour

1/3 cup rice flour

2 tablespoons melted butter

1/2 cup whipping cream

1/2 teaspoon baking soda

1/2 teaspoon cream of tartar

1/4 to 1/2 cup of water

Into a large bowl, sift flour with baking soda and cream of tartar. With a wooden spoon add butter and blend. Stir in cream and enough water to make a soft dough.

Turn out on a well-floured pastry board. Sprinkle lightly with flour. Knead dough 2 minutes. Divide dough in half. Shape each half into a ball. Flatten each ball into a 1/2 inch thick circle. Slice each circle into quarters.

Sprinkle a baking sheet with cornmeal or other flour. Place scones on sheet about 1 inch apart. Bake at 475° for 15 to 20 minutes. Makes 8 scones.

SUMMARY

In this book I have tried to explain the many ways that we upset our body chemistry and also the many ways that we can enhance our chemistry. Your health is up to you. We live in a polluted world. Our water is not as clean as it should be. The air we breathe has many chemicals. The food we eat has lost some of its nutritional value due to the deficient soil. And the chemicals we use to overcome that soil depletion, as well as the often long shipping and shelf life only make things worse. Much of this is out of our control, but there is so much you can control to keep your immune system as strong as possible so that you can handle the outside influences. Remember that what you do on a daily basis with your body — what you eat, how you feel, where you live and work, what you say and what you do — is so much more important than outside pollutants.

I hope I have helped you to understand your basic health and how you can create a healthy body by balancing your body chemistry. After years of not being healthy, I have created my health — I feel better than I did when I was 20 years old. In our society with all its temptations, I have to continually make choices as to whether I will upset my body chemistry or not by my food intake, my actions, thoughts, and feelings. Our life is a process, one of making choices, evaluating and re-evaluating; learning from mistakes and moving on. I hope this book has taught you that you can choose to be healthy. The biggest secret of natural healing is this: stop doing things to throw your chemistry out of balance, and your body will heal itself.

ABOUT THE AUTHOR

This book is written by nutritionist Dr. Nancy Appleton, author of the books *Lick the Sugar Habit* and *Healthy Bones*, and the audio series *The Balanced Body Secret*. Dr. Appleton is in private practice and also conducts lectures and workshops around the country, teaching people how to take charge of their health through balancing their body chemistry.

Order Information for Body Chemistry Kit

There is an easy method to determine if your calcium and phosphorus are in the right ratio. The test works by measuring the amount of calcium in the urine. In the privacy of your home, you can test to see if you are secreting too much calcium, the right amount of calcium, or too little calcium. Since calcium only works in relationship to phosphorus, this test tells whether the phosphorus is too low for the calcium present or if the phosphorus is in the right relation to the calcium.

If the calcium and phosphorus are in the right relationship, then the rest of the minerals are in the right relationship. When the minerals are in the right relationship, the enzymes can function optimally and the body is more apt to stay healthy and also heal.

The kit includes solution for more than 250 tests, two test tubes, and eye dropper, a brush for cleaning test tubes, and a 28-page instruction booklet, How to Monitor Your Basic Health by Bruce Pacetti, D.D.S. and Nancy Appleton, Ph.D. This booklet contains a section on what upsets body chemistry, suggestions on how to balance body chemistry, food plans, and a section on how to test for food allergies. Also included is pH paper to test for acid-alkalinity of the saliva and urine.

1 kit	$20.00
Shipping	$2.00
Sales tax (California residents only)	$1.65

Send name, address, and check payable to:

Nancy Appleton, Ph.D.
P.O. Box 3083
Santa Monica, Ca. 90403-3083

GLOSSARY

ADRENAL GLANDS: Two glands in the upper back part of the abdomen (atop the kidneys) which produce and secrete vital hormones.

ALLERGEN (Antigen): A foreign protein, as in a food, bacteria, or virus, that stimulates a specific immune response when introduced into the body.

ANTIBODY: A substance capable of producing immunity to a specific germ or virus; our bodies also form antibodies to undigested food in the bloodstream.

AMENORRHEA: Failure of menstruation.

ANTERIOR PITUITARY GLAND: The front portion of the pituitary gland located at the base of the skull; it produces important hormones such as growth hormone.

ARTHRITIS: Inflammation of a joint or tissue surrounding the joint.

BASOPHIL: White blood cell.

BODY CHEMISTRY: The functioning of the body systems which depend upon the body's chemical balance, which depends upon balanced mineral relationships.

CANDIDA ALBICANS: A fungus, which can be local (as in vaginal infections) or systemic.

CAPILLARIES: Very small blood vessels; it is from the capillaries that nourishment is fed directly to the tissues.

DEGENERATIVE DISEASE: A deterioration of tissue with loss of function and eventual destruction of the particular tissue cells.

ENDOCRINE GLAND: A gland, such as pituitary, thyroid, and adrenal, which secretes its hormones into the blood stream.

ENDOMETRIAL CANCER: Cancer of the mucous membrane lining the uterine cavity.

ENZYME: A protein that accelerates specific chemical reactions but does not itself undergo any change during the reaction; a biochemical catalyst; digestive enzymes are produced by glands and organs to break down complex carbohydrates into simple sugars, fats or lipids into fatty acids; glycerol, glycerides, and protein into amino acids.

EOSINOPHIL: White blood cells which increase in number when a person has an allergic reaction or when there is an invasion of the body by a parasite.

ESTROGEN: The hormone responsible for the development and maintenance of female sexual characteristics and reproductive function in women; the ovaries produce estrogen in women and the testes produce small amounts of estrogen in men.

GENETICS: The science dealing with heredity.

GLAND: An organ which manufactures a chemical which will be utilized elsewhere; if this chemical secretion goes into the bloodstream, the gland belongs to the endocrine system (such as the pancreas); if the chemical secretes through a duct (tube) to surrounding tissues, it is an exocrine gland (such as the salivary glands).

GLUCOSE: A simple sugar; the end product of the digestion of starch, sucrose, maltose, and lactose; it provides most of the energy for the cells of the body.

GOUT: A type of arthritis or inflammation about the joint caused by excess uric acid in the blood; attacks occur suddenly and are accompanied by great pain; the big toe is a frequent site.

HOMEOSTASIS: The state of equilibrium (balance between opposing pressures) in the body with respect to various functions and to the chemical compositions of the fluids and tissues, e.g., pH, temperature, heart rate, blood pressure, water content, blood sugar; this is accomplished in large part by the hormones.

HORMONE: A chemical produced by a gland, secreted into the blood, and affecting the function of distant cells or organs.

HYDROCHLORIC ACID (HCl): Hydrogen chloride, an acid secreted by the cells lining the stomach; helps the digestion of food.

HYPERTENSION: High blood pressure.

HYPERGLYCEMIA: Excessive sugar in the blood.

HYPOGLYCEMIA: Too little sugar in the blood.

HYPOTHALAMUS: The master gland of the neuroendocrine system; controls the brain, the pituitary's production, and the release of its own hormone.

IMMUNE SYSTEM: The body's system that defends us against disease, composed primarily of white blood cells (the bone marrow, the thymus gland, and the lymph tissue are prominent in activating the immune system.)

IMMUNOGLOBULIN: Antibody produced in the lymphatic cells to combat infections or other invading substances subdivided into five classes: lgG, lgA, lgE, lgM, and lgF.

LIPID: Fat.

LIPOPROTEIN: Complex compounds of lipids and carbohydrates.

METABOLISM: The process by which foods are transformed into basic elements that can be utilized by the body for energy or growth.

OSTEOARTHRITIS: A form of arthritis associated with bone and cartilage degeneration.

OSTEOPOROSIS: Loss of bone or skeletal tissue, producing brittleness or softness of bone.

PANCREAS: An endocrine gland in upper portion of the abdomen which secretes the hormones insulin and glucagon into the bloodstream, and secretes digestive enzymes and bicarbonate into the intestine.

PARATHYROID GLAND: One of four small endocrine glands located in the neck; secretes the hormone which controls calcium and phosphorus metabolism.

PASTEURIZATION: The heating of milk products, wine, fruit juices, etc., for about 30 minutes at 154.4° F whereby the living bacteria are destroyed but the flavor is protected; the molecular structure of the food changes.

PERIODONTAL DISEASE: A disease of the tissues, including the gums, immediately surrounding the teeth (pyorrhea).

pH: A symbol denoting acidity or alkalinity; a solution of pH 7 is neutral, below 7 is acidic, above 7 is alkaline.

PHAGOCYTE: White blood cell which can eat or destroy foreign matter or bacteria.

PITUITARY: An endocrine gland in the base of the brain; secretes several hormones and seems to control the secretions of other glands such as the thyroid and adrenals.

PMS (Premenstrual Syndrome): A period of tension, bloating, irritability, headaches, food allergies, nervousness, and swelling and pain in the breasts seen in some women for a few days prior to menstruation.

POSTPITUITARY GLAND (Posterior Pituitary): A portion of the pituitary which secretes hormones such as an antidiuretic hormone.

SINUSITIS: Inflammation of one of the sinuses about the nose.

SUGAR: Sucrose; a disaccharide consisting of glucose and fructose found in all foods, even fat and protein.

THYROID: Endocrine gland located in front of the neck; regulates body metabolism; secretes a hormone known as thyroxin.

BIBLIOGRAPHY

Abraham, Gary E., "Nutritional Factors in the Etiology of the Premenstrual Tension Syndrome." Journal of Reproductive Medicine. 28:7, July 1983.

Allen, L.H., Bloch, R.S., and Bloch, G.P. "The Reduction of Renal Calcium Absorption in Man by Consumption of Dietary Proteins." Journal of Nutrition.109 (1979):1345-1350.

Allen, Michael. "Poor Physical Fitness Is Linked to Premature Death in a Study." Wall Street Journal. Nov. 3, 1989.

Appleton, Nancy. *Healthy Bones*. Garden City Park, New York: Avery Publishing, 1991.

Appleton, Nancy. *Lick the Sugar Habit*. Garden City Park, New York: Avery Publishing, 1983.

Ayalon, J., Simkin, A., Leichter, I., and Raefmann, S. "Dynamic Bone Loading Exercises of Post Menopausal Women." Archives of Physical Medical Rehabilitation. 68, no. 5 (May 1987):280-283.

Bailey, D.A., Martin, A.D., Houstin, C.S., and Howie, J.L. "Physical Activity, Nutrition, Bone Density, and Osteoporosis." Australian Journal of Science Medicine in Sports. Sept. 3-7, 1986.

Barnes, Broda, and Galton, Laurence. *Hypothyroidism: The Unsuspected Illness.* New York: Thomas Y. Crowell Co., 1976.

Barrow, M. "Hypothermia." Natural Healing Newsletter. 3:26,4.

Berger, Stuart M. *Dr. Berger's Immune Power Diet.* New York: New American Library, 1985.

Beverly, L.N. "Shine a Light on Depression and Get Rid of Those Winter Blues." Natural Healing Newsletter. 3,30:7.

Bland, Jeffrey, Ph.D. *Medical Applications of Clinical Nutrition.* New Canaan, Connecticut. Keats Publishing, 1983.

Breneman, J.C. *Basics of Food Allergy.* Springfield, Illinois: Charles C. Thomas, 1978.

Buttram, H.E. "Overuse of Antibiotics and the Need for Alternatives." *Townsend Letter for Doctors.* Nov. 1991, pp. 867-872.

Caldwell, Betsie, *et al.*, eds. *Health: A Concern for Every American.* Wylie, Texas: Information Plus, 1991.

Chaplan, Abraham. "PMS Syndrome: Let's Bring Women Out of the 19th Century." Nutritional Consultant. July 1984, pp. 46-48.

Cousins, Norman. *Anatomy of an Illness.* New York: Bantam, 1983.

Crook, William G. *The Yeast Connection.* Jackson, Tennessee: Professional Books, 1984.

Darlington, L.G., Ramsey, N.W., and Mansfield, J.R. "Placebo-Controlled Blind Study of Dietary Manipulation Therapy in Rheumatoid Arthritis." Lancet. Feb. 6, 1986, pp. 236-38.

"Electricity and Cancer," Bottom Line. August 15, 1991.

Fisher, Irving. "The Influence of Flesh Eating on Endurance." Yale Medical Journal. 13 (5):205-221, 1907.

Forman, Robert. *How to Control Your Allergies*. New York: Larchmont Books, 1979.

Foster, Carol, et al., eds. *Woman's Changing Role*. Wylie, Texas: Information Plus, 1991.

Friedman, Howard. "Open Mind." *Longevity*. November 1990, p.26.

"Fighting Disease with Exercise: Health After 50." *John Hopkins Medical Letter*: 3,5, July 1991.

Gittleman, Ann Louise. *Super Nutrition for Women*. New York: Bantam Books, 1991.

Howell, Edward. *Enzyme Nutrition*. Garden City Park, New York: Avery Publishing, 1985.

Kamen, Betty, and Kamen, Si. *Osteoporosis: What It Is, How to Prevent It, How to Stop It*. New York: Pinnacle Books, Inc., 1984.

Kaslow, Arthur L., and Miles, Richard B. *Freedom from Chronic Disease*. Los Angeles, California: J.P. Tarcher, 1979.

Kenton, Leslie, and Kenton, Susan. *Raw Energy*. New York: Warner Books, 1984.

Krooh, L. "Periodontal Disease in Dogs and Man." Adv. Vet. Sci. Comp. Med.. 20:171-190, 1976.

Jackson, J.A., et al.. "Aluminum from a Coffee Pot." Lancet. 1989, 1:781-782.

Lehninger, Albert L. *Principles of Biochemistry*. New York: Worth Publishers, Inc., 1987.

Levitsky, David, and Obarzanek, Eva. "How to Do Everything Right." New York Board Room Reports, 1989.

Lewis, Juanita L., and Lauroso, Nicola Michael. "PMS (Premenstrual Syndrome) Can be Prevented and Cured." The Living Health Bulletin. 2:17 & 18, 1984, pp. 1-13.

Ludeman, Kate, and Henderson, Louise. *Do-It-Yourself Allergy Analysis Handbook.* New Canaan, Connecticut: Keats Publishing, Inc., 1979.

Mackarness, Richard. *Eating Dangerously: The Hazards of Hidden Allergies.* New York and London: Harcourt Brace Jovanovich, 1976.

Mandell, Marshall, and Scanlon, Lynne Waller. *Dr. Mandell's 5-Day Allergy Relief System.* New York: Thomas Y. Crowell, 1979.

Mason, Jim, and Enger, Peter. *Animal Factories.* New York: Crown Publishers, 1980.

May, Margaret Whitney. "Shaping Up". Wall Street Journal. Jan. 23, 1991., p.2.

Mayes, Katherine. *Osteoporosis: Brittle Bones and the Calcium Crisis.* Santa Barbara, California: Pennant Books, 1986.

Mervyn, Len. *Minerals and Your Health.* New Canaan, Connecticut: Keats Publishing, 1981.

Notelovitz, Morris, and Ware, Marsha. *Stand Tall.* New York: Bantam Books, 1985.

Page, Melvin. Degeneration — Regeneration. St. Petersburg Beach, Florida: Nutritional Development, 1949.

Page, Melvin E. and Abrams, H. Leon. Health and Disease. St. Petersburg, Florida: Page Foundation, 1971.

Page, Melvin E. Body Chemistry in Health and Disease. St. Petersburg, Florida: Nutritional Development.

Page, Melvin, and Abrams, H. Leon. *Your Body Is Your Best Doctor.* New Canaan, Connecticut: Keats Publishing, 1972.

"Painting Your Walls Could Harm You." New England Journal of Medicine. Oct. 18, 1990, 232,16:1096.

Philpott, William H., and Kalita, Dwight K. *Brain Allergies.* New Canaan, Connecticut: Keats Publishing.

Philpott, William H., and Kalita, Dwight K. *Victory Over Diabetes.* New Canaan, Connecticut. Keats Publishing, 1983.

"Poisoned People: Detoxing Body Tissue." Longevity. March 1991, 84.

Randolph, Theron G., and Moss, Ralph W. *An Alternative Approach to Allergies.* New York: Bantam Books, 1980.

Reddy, B. "Nutrition and Its Relation to Cancer". Advances in Cancer Research, 32:237, 1980.

"Researchers Suspect that Electric Blankets Increase Risk of Cancer." Natural Healing Newsletter. 3:3.

Rinkel, H.J., Randolph, T.G., and Zeller, M. *Food Allergy.* Norwalk, Connecticut: New England Foundation of Allergic and Environmental Diseases (reprinted 1951).

Robbins, John. *Diet for a New America.* Walpole, NH: Stillpoint Publishing, 1987.

Scheer, James F. "Health Notes." Health Freedom News. Oct. 1990, p. 32.

Schell, O. Modern Meat. Vintage Books, Random House, 1985, p. 254.

"Second Hand Smoke." Natural Healing Newsletter. 3:26,4.

Siblerud, R.L. "The Relationship Between Mercury From Dental Amalgam and Oral Cavity Health." Annals of Dentistry. Winter, 1990.

Simmson, Maria, and Hulman, Joan Raltner. *The Complete University Medical Diet.* New York: Rawson Associates, 1983.

Stedman's Medical Dictionary. Baltimore, Maryland: The Williams & Wilkins Co., 1979.

Taeuber, Cynthia. *Statistical Handbook on Women in America.* Phoenix, Arizona: Onyx Press, 1991.

Tofler, Alvin. *Future Shock.* New York: Random House, 1970.

"Who Outlives Whom: Solid Citizens or Wackos?" Longevity. Sept. 1991.

"Young Women, Weight and Stress." Bottom Line. Researchers at Tufts University. Oct. 30, 1990, p. 9.

INDEX

ABOUT RUDRA PRESS

We hope you enjoy *Secrets of Natural Healing with Food: Wellness and Body Chemistry*. Rudra Press strives to publish the finest books, audios and videos on health and healing, spirituality, and hatha yoga. Practical, powerful, simple, and clear, our products are designed to meet the needs of modern life and to support our customers in their quest for personal growth. Increased health, inner balance, and well-being are just a few of the many benefits contained in Rudra Press's products. Of related interest:

Books

Yoga for Body, Breath, and Mind (revised) by A.G. Mohan

Healing Imagery and Music by Carol Bush, L.C.S.W.

The Breath of God by Swami Chetanananda

A Healer's Journey by Sree Chakravarti

Food Facts, by Rachel Brooks M.D.

Stretch and Surrender: A Guide to Yoga, Health, and Relaxation for People in Recovery by Annalisa Cunningham, M.A.

Audios

The Balanced Body Secret by Nancy Appleton, Ph.D.

The SMART Way to Relax by Arlin Brown, M.D.

For more information on Rudra Press's complete line of products or to request a free catalog, please call toll free 1-800-876-7798 or fax 1-800-394-6286.

Rudra Press
P.O. Box 13390
Portland, OR 97213